PSYCHIATRY - THEORY, APPLICATIONS AND TREATMENTS

FORENSIC PSYCHIATRY AND ETHICAL APPROACHES IN LEGAL ISSUES

PSYCHIATRY - THEORY, APPLICATIONS AND TREATMENTS

Additional books and e-books in this series can be found on Nova's website under the Series tab.

PSYCHIATRY - THEORY, APPLICATIONS AND TREATMENTS

FORENSIC PSYCHIATRY AND ETHICAL APPROACHES IN LEGAL ISSUES

NURSEN TURAN YURTSEVER
EDITOR

nova
Medicine & Health
New York

Additional color graphics may be available in the e-book version of this book.

Library of Congress Cataloging-in-Publication Data

ISBN: 978-1-53619-530-9

Published by Nova Science Publishers, Inc. † New York

CONTENTS

PREFACE

I hope that this book will be a useful resource for those working in forensic psychiatry settings or work with offender populations when it comes to ethical decisions faced in their clinical practice.

This book consists of ten chapters. The first chapter puts in the current perspective of forensic psychiatry and its relation with medical ethics.The second chapter focuses on criminal responsibility and legal capacity. The subsequent chapters focus on specialized areas of forensic psychiatry practice that come with ethical issues. The last two chapters of this book focuses on forensic child psychiatry in relation to child custody and interview with child victim. Chapters in this book includes cases which are fictional, not real, but emphasis is made on the events that may be encountered in real life.

To list moral dilemmas that clinicians face in their everyday clinical practice was not possible in this book as it would be impossible to debate all of them in one book.

I would like to thank all authors for their excellent contributions to this book and also to thank Prof. Aysegul Demirhan Erdemir, Prof. Salih Yasar Ozden as reviewers of this book.

I would like to thank Nova Science Publishers in delivering this book.

I would like to thank my son, Alper and my husband, Selcuk for their understanding during my hardworking process.

Nursen Turan Yurtsever
31, December, 2020,
Istanbul

In: Forensic Psychiatry …
Editor: Nursen Turan Yurtsever
ISBN: 978-1-53619-530-9

Chapter 1

CURRENT FORENSIC PSYCHIATRY AND MEDICAL ETHICS

Nursen Turan Yurtsever*, MD
Forensic Medicine Department,
Marmara University, School of Medicine,
Istanbul, Turkey

ABSTRACT

The action of crime and the interaction of individuals with a crime on a personal and societal basis constitute the topic of forensic psychiatry. Despite the fact that the primary purpose of the forensic psychiatrist is to make an evaluation of the patient so as to respond to the questions that are being asked by the court, medical ethical rules have to be in place in all applications of the forensic psychiatrist. Such activities are administered by way of regulations that are formed within organizations and through the activities of professional bodies and related organizations that include experts in each country. All the general rules that apply for medical ethics apply for applications of psychiatry as well. According to what is stated in the Declaration of the World Medical Association, the physician should

* Corresponding Author's E-mail: nursenturan@yahoo.com.

first consider the advantage of his patient. However, when crimes such as sexual assault, murder or child abuse that are perpetrated against humanity are being hidden, or when the perpetrators are protected or hidden, the situation does not coincide with ethical principles.

INTRODUCTION TO FORENSIC PSYCHIATRY

The action of a crime and the interaction of individuals with the crime on a personal and societal basis constitute the topic of forensic psychiatry. To detect the impact of a crime on a person as well as the contribution of the psychological state of the person to the action of the crime, and then the evaluation of the legal sanctions and psychiatric phenomena in this context together with the psychiatric treatment of people that are hospitalized or who were arrested in a forensic psychiatry hospital are the areas of occupation of forensic psychiatry (Niveau and Welle 2018; Völlm et al. 2018).

Forensic psychiatry is a topic that concerns many occupations and branches of science, such as law, medicine, psychiatry, psychology, criminology, toxicology, public health and social services (Niveau and Welle 2018).

The General Medical Council (2004) and specialties in medicine such as the American Psychiatric Association (1995) and the Royal College of Psychiatrists (2000) arrange their professional organizations and applications by way of ethical rules. As a result, a path is followed with specific rules in terms of professional education and so that the application and emergence of chaos is hindered within the field. Furthermore, many societies of specialization have arranged application guidelines for forensic psychiatry as a subfield and have formed articles relating to ethics (Niveau and Welle 2018; Völlm et al. 2018).

Likewise, there are discussions in the sense of specialization and quality relating to individuals who may become experts. Such activities are administered by way of regulations that are formed within organizations and through the activities of the professional bodies and related organizations that include experts in each country (Fox and Levy 2013; Völlm et al. 2018; Simon and Gold 2010).

Throughout the world, the education period that applies for forensic psychiatrists are changing; however, psychiatry specialists take board examinations after a 4-year psychiatry education on average. After the board examinations, they complete a rigorous one-year, full-time, accredited post-residency fellowship in forensic psychiatry and take the board examination again. There are very few official forensic psychiatrists that pass board examinations (Fox and Levy 2013). On the other hand, in Turkey, like in many European countries, no forensic psychiatry education exists after the psychiatry education; the psychiatry specialists that officiate in the field of forensic medicine do a job as a forensic psychiatrist. The councils that are formed with the attendance of specialists from the fields of forensic medicine, neurology and psychology together with the child and adolescent psychiatrists in the field of forensic psychiatry render expert service to the courts.

The American Academy of Psychiatry and the Law (AAPL) published the Ethical Guidelines for the Practice of Forensic Psychiatry. The Ethical Guidelines for the Practice of Forensic Psychiatry has a statement in section V, that "expertise in the practice of forensic psychiatry should be claimed only in areas of actual knowledge, skills, training, and experience" (Arboleda-Florez 2006; Simon and Gold 2010).

Despite the fact that definite clear limitations are drawn in the sense of education and experience, many physicians who do not bear the qualifications render expert service in the field of forensic psychiatry. The attorneys and some psychiatrists do not somehow pay attention to the distinction of roles between the psychiatrist that gives the treatment and one who is an expert. Whether many psychiatrists who officiate as an expert comprehend the mission and vision of forensic psychiatry is an additional topic that arouses curiosity since the approach of a clinical psychiatrist and that of a forensic psychiatrist actually differ in the sense of purpose and application (Fox and Levy 2013; Niveau and Welle 2018). Within the scope of forensic psychiatry, which bears very different dynamics than clinical psychiatry in the sense of the relationship with the patient, it is possible to make comparisons.

The psychiatrist or the therapist who assumes the treatment of their patient has to believe in their patient and to firstly treat their pain. On the other hand, a psychiatrist who has the role of an expert person is obliged to approach what the patient has told them with doubt, to test the accuracy and to examine it. The treatment of the patient is already ensured or generally continued by another physician. The mission of the physician as an expert is to obtain the facts and to submit them to the judicial authority (Appelbaum 1997; Niveau and Welle 2018; Fox and Levy 2013; Völlm et al. 2018). He has to provide a health service for the patient as an ethical must in emergency cases, however, in the sense of continuity of treatment, the fact that the treatment of the patient is continued by another physician is more ethical and appropriate. In terms of the evaluation of a patient, it is difficult that a psychiatrist who officiates as an expert for the court to establish an efficient patient physician relationship as a therapist during the treatment of the same patient (Fox and Levy 2013; Völlm et al. 2018; Simon and Gold 2010).

While the therapist considers what the patient said and what he envisaged in his mind as accurate and that is reflected in his report, an experienced forensic psychiatrist will state the closeness of what the patient said to the facts together with the possible diagnosis and outcomes in detail as based on evidence in his report (Appelbaum 1997; Fox and Levy 2013; Völlm et al. 2018)).

For instance, when a kleptomaniac patient is referred to a therapist to have a report issued by the court, most possibly, the therapist states that the person perpetrated the crime of theft by reason of his disease. However, an experienced forensic psychiatrist interrogates the quality of the incident of theft. For instance, relating to whether it is a petty theft like stealing a worthless item from the supermarket or else a major crime like stealing a large amount of money from a bank, whether the crime had been planned beforehand, the previous types of crimes that the person perpetrated, the sensation of the person before, during or after the crime. He carries out detailed examinations on many matters and collects evidence regarding them. On the other hand, at the end of his report, he states his probable decisions by way of justifying them based on evidence. The report that the forensic psychiatrist issues becomes well-qualified at the end of his education as well as experience acquired in this field. A well-qualified report both covers the necessity of the attorney at the phase of decision-making and assures justice both from the perspective of the victim and the offender (Appelbaum 1997).

The peculiarities that have been deemed as common on an international basis for proficiency may be assessed under the title of specialization, knowledge, skills, education and experience (Simon and Gold 2010).

A specialization or education in an upper branch may require that the forensic psychiatrist possesses special knowledge and experience for the qualifications of an expert person in various fields (the Violations of Human Rights, the Abuse of Children, etc.) (American Academy of Psychiatry and the Law).

At the time of making a forensic psychiatric evaluation, it may be required to join together the perspectives of many disciplines. Therefore, at the time of examining a case that became a matter of forensic psychiatry, it may be of benefit that the incident is divided into phases in the sense of establishing a more objective approach (Völlm et al. 2018). It is significant to establish a schedule that includes before the forensic case, the forensic case itself and after the forensic case and to become cognizant of factors such as persons, environment and other contributing factors and to gather the information and to make effort to hinder any gap remaining while forming a picture of the case (Turan Yurtsever 2019).

Before the Forensic Case: Facts to be determined include the background of the person, the physical and psychological state of health so as to make an evaluation of near or distant past, the experiences that he had relating to the forensic case, the interactions he built with the present persons as part of the incident, the place of the incident and the nearness to the person/persons, the opinions, plans and emotional reactions of the person relating to the forensic case (Turan Yurtsever 2019).

The Process of the Forensic Case: Facts to be determined include the date and hour when the case started, for how long it continued, the reasons that incited it, the actions that the person carried out relating to the case during the process, his emotional reactions and what he said, the way he put an end to the case and how long it took, the outcome of the case or the harms that emerged, the people that were in the surroundings at the time of the case and their interactions relating to the case, the findings of the place of the incident, videos, photographs, charts and alike (Turan Yurtsever 2019; Igoumenou 2020).

After the Forensic Case: Research is carried out relating to the existence of the psychological and physical findings that have developed with the person, the regret, anger, relief and similar emotions that the case caused with the person or the lack of any emotional reactions, the comment of the person relating to the case, the comments of the people and incident witnesses that were present around the person, the behavioral changes that developed with the person after the case, the changes that developed in the business and social areas, the impacts that the case had upon the economic assets of the person, and the presence of similar actions that the person carried out after the case (Turan Yurtsever 2019).

As part of the forensic psychiatry, to do a good quality interrogation relating to the case is as significant as determining the states of psychological and physical health. In order to differentiate whether the person is liable for the actions relating to the case, it is necessary to establish a bond between the physical and psychological reactions that he made relating to the case (Völlm et al. 2018). An evaluation has to be made relating to the inability of any chronological ordering as part of the cases that the person caused, the lack of emergence of logical meaning of the actions that he did relating to the relevant case or the lack of a physical and psychological advantage of the person relating to the case, the lack of planning relating to the case and whether the person bears any psychological disorders relating to the case (Igoumenou 2020).

While doing an integrated anamnesis of a psychiatry patient, the information that are special to the person includes stories of the family anamnesis starting from childhood, education, professional or school life, social life, pregnancy and sexual life. While obtaining such information, the psychiatrist becomes cognizant of very special information that are peculiar to the patient, such as previous life stories, experiences, expectations for the future, dreams and wishes (Cetin 2019). If the patient does not rely on the psychiatrist, he may not provide enough information or may give inadequate information as a result of which correct diagnosis and treatment may not be applied. However, the purpose in forensic psychiatry is to receive the most accurate information relating to the patient and to make a response to the forensic questions (Simon and Gold 2010). Therefore, in order for the forensic psychiatrist to obtain the necessary information from their patient, a single meeting may not be adequate. Particularly, adequate time becomes necessary for repeated examinations and tests for detecting a mental disease (Gelder and et al. 2006; Völlm et al. 2018).

Despite the fact that forensic psychiatry comes to mind at the first glance as the common point of psychiatry and areas of the law, when we gather these two different areas together, more complicated headings emerge in terms of both the topic and the application (Sen P et al. 2007). In this field, which concerns many areas of discipline and for which the borders cannot be drawn, misunderstanding, confusion in the mind, complications and even abuses are unavoidable such that medical ethics become guiding in such situations. Under hospital conditions where the patients surrender themselves to the physicians entirely and where they share even their most private issues, the application of ethics gains a high importance for protection of both the patient and the physician (Cetin B 2019). Ethics is called medical ethics if used in a medical sense and together with medical applications.

Medical Ethics for Forensic Psychiatry

The forensic psychiatrist is obliged to apply the traditional principles of ethics in his work. However, in some cases, the forensic rules may be contradictory to such principles. In these cases, the forensic psychiatrist must decide what has priority (American Academy of Psychiatry and the Law; Arboleda-Florez 2006; Simon and Gold 2010).

Throughout the world, physicians deal with patients as individuals in addition to protecting personal rights, ensuring the confidentiality of information that is shared with inclusion of the disease, providing empathy relating to the case and improving the disease condition. The physician's occupation acts in a way focused on human beings on a personal basis with the decisions that they make and the applications that they carry out (Appelbaum1997; Cetin 2019). However, Should the physician keep the personal information and the state of health of his patient superior to the society if no common denominator with the society is at hand?

The behavior of occupational professionalism is open to many comments in cases of conflict of rights and requires that physicians interpret the ethical content to some extent on a philosophical basis (Appelbaum 1997). However, as we gather comments and perspectives that differ, how should a true approach become apparent that does not push the ethical borders of the physician's job and, most importantly, that does not interrupt the relationship between the patient and the physician?

All the general rules that apply with medical ethics apply for applications of psychiatry as well. For example, medical codes of practice throughout the world contain an absolute prohibition against sexual relationships with a patient. The therapist should not state his religious beliefs and personal value judgments to his patient and should not impose them on him. For instance, a physician should not make statements regarding a woman who wishes to have an abortion done by reason of an unwanted pregnancy, for instance that she should not get this abortion done due to religious reasons (Gelder and et al. 2006).

Despite being appointed by the court, the initial and the most important task of the clinician is not to cause harm to his patient (Niveau and Welle 2018; Völlm et al. 2018; Taborda and Arboleda-Flórez 2006). This is particularly a very significant ethical problem in countries where death sentences are in force. In order for the death sentence to be put into practice, it has to be determined by the forensic psychiatrist whether the convict is sane or not. How could a physician issue a healthy report when he is cognizant of the fact that the person that he has examined will get killed legally by reason of the healthy mental report that he issues? Then, is it ethical for him to issue an untrue report in order to save the life of his patient? Both of these do not constitute a true approach. Just as the patient bears the right to reject the examination or select his physician, the physician bears the right to reject carrying out an examination by reason of ethical reasons as well. In cases that conflict with ethical principles or that hinder the physician from acting neutrally or carrying out his occupation as is due, his rejection of carrying out an examination will be the most proper approach and also he should make his action known to his professional organization (Arboleda-Florez 2006).

As stated in the joint declaration of the World Medical Association and many physician's associations, for physicians to attend to any tortures and/or any harmful behaviors giving pain to human beings, or that they provide information, material or support to such behaviors are by no means acceptable behavior (Taborda and Arboleda-Flórez 2006; Niveau and Welle 2018).

Four major ethical principles are respect for autonomy, beneficence (benefit to patients), non-maleficence (not to harm) and justice (Sen P etal. 2007; Eastman et al. 2018).

General Medical Ethics

Despite the fact that the primary purpose of the forensic psychiatrist is to make an evaluation of the patient so as to respond to questions that are being asked by the court, medical ethical rules must have a place in all applications of the forensic psychiatrist (Appelbaum1997; Niveau and Welle 2018; Völlm et al. 2018). The physician does not discriminate among his patients by reason of race, religion, language, ethnicity, gender, age or other differences. The physician gives respect to his patient for any reason that the patient came for an examination (American Academy of Psychiatry and the Law; Völlm et al. 2018). He accepts that his patient bears personal rights like selecting his physician and does not impose pressure on him.

The forensic psychiatrist obtains information that he acquired from his patient based on his impartial observations and what is needed in order for him to issue a report. The forensic psychiatrist does not make any effort to grasp the private information of the patient that remains outside the topic for the sake of his personal curiosity. He interprets to his colleagues that are in the position of experts for the integrity of the report and with the information related to the topics that have been asked (Robertson 2000; Simon and Gold 2010).

The Hippocratic tradition of primum non nocere (first do not harm) still is the rule of the profession to which physicians give an oath after graduation (Taborda and Arboleda-Flórez 2006). Physicians bear a similar responsibility before both their patients and all the health personnel including their colleagues with whom they collaborate while they are working. Therefore, they are liable to work in harmony with the health personnel with whom they collaborate and other similar organizational teams, to take true steps that are required by the profession, to envisage the probable harmful steps and act prudently beforehand. The physician has to know the society around him as well as his social circles. As a result, he will be able to interpret the information provided by patients coming to him and will handle his patient as a single individual, taking measures for their best advantage (American Academy of Psychiatry and the Law).

Case 1

As part of an interview with a girl who was brought by her father by reason of her psychiatric problems, in case the girl says all of a sudden that she incurred sexual abuse by her boyfriend, it bears importance to take measures that conform to the condition of the girl. For instance, to tell about this situation directly to the father who comes from a family with customs that may lead to damaging his daughter by saying that she had sexual intercourse as a matter of chastity may lead to serious incidents. In this case, the physician has to take preventive measures such as providing the security of the girl in the first place and then to make a judicial announcement of the case. The physician additionally has to know the addresses and phone numbers to contact the relevant institutions. He has to be cognizant of whether the child will firstly be referred to social services, how the persons concerned will be reached or what means of communication will be made use of in order to give information to the courthouse or the prosecutor. If the girl does not give clear information or a case of abuse is a matter of doubt, a path may be followed such as calling the girl for an interview once again and asking for a consultation from specialist physicians that officiate in the relevant fields.

If it is not possible to avoid complications with treatment of the disease, the treatment with the least complication and the solution of the situation with the least damage to the patient in case of an encounter should be provided (American Academy of Psychiatry and the Law).

Informed Consent

However, the psychiatrist should be sure that the information relating to his patient will not be transmitted to unauthorized people. Ensuring the security of the information constitutes the task of the physician (Niveau and Welle 2018; Appelbaum 1997; Taborda and Arboleda-Flórez 2006). On the other hand, keeping information that is recorded as part of the health system and closing it to the access of others is under the responsibility of the manager of the health organization and the data processing employees (Cetin 2019).

The psychiatrist should be informed on practices of law that apply in the region where he officiates and should not make promises that he can't keep to his patient. Likewise, he should have the attitude of gaining true and correct information from his patient and providing it to his patient. He should determine whether the patient is an inpatient or outpatient and should arrange the approach of treatment accordingly. Therefore, he should obtain the contact information of the prosecutor or the judge that had referred the forensic patient, should grasp the necessary details and should determine the method that is appropriate for the evaluation, monitoring and treatment process for the forensic patient (American Academy of Psychiatry and the Law).

Consent relating to a forensic case should be received before the examination, as with each patient. For instance, as the person enters the examination room for the first time, after making an introduction in the form of "I am Dr. Suzan, my specialty is psychiatry, I have been appointed by the court for the purpose of examining and evaluating you," they should continue with, “I’m a physician but not the physician who will treat you” and they should ask whether the person is cognizant of why they have come for an examination(American Academy of Psychiatry and the Law; Taborda and Arboleda-Flórez 2006; Simon and Gold 2010).

Information should be provided before the examination relating to the reason why the examination is being done, what kind of an examination will be given and for what purpose the information obtained in the course of the examination will be put to use or to whom the information will be transmitted in detail, taking into consideration the age, intelligence, education and mental state of the person. They should evaluate whether the person has comprehended the reason for the examination and for what purpose the information to be obtained will be put to use (American Academy of Psychiatry and the Law; Taborda and Arboleda-Flórez 2006; Simon and Gold 2010).

If the person continues with the interview or does not reject the examination after obtaining this information, it will be accepted that their consent has been received.

Despite the fact that it is a forensic case, pushing the person for an examination does not coincide with ethical principles. Moreover, no definitive information can be obtained as a result of examination done by force. In cases where the person does not have to give consent, the person making the evaluation should receive verbal consent and should also state this in his evaluation. In cases where the interview is being recorded by video, the consent of the patient should be received for the video recording and as a result, it may be easily determined with the record that the patient has given consent (Fox and Levy 2013). The way of recording of the consent as part of the one-to-one interview of the patient with the physician may be in a verbal and/or written manner. As part of forensic psychiatric examinations, because a nurse or health official in general does not participate in the examination, it would be a benefit to have an audio and/or video recording.

Respect for Autonomy

In cases where the patient cannot give consent, it may be adequate to receive consent from a relative as his guardian. However, in cases where the reliability of the statement of the person is questionable, it will not be adequate to receive consent for cases referred by the court (Simon and Gold 2010). In lieu of this, if the person rejects the examination, this information should be recorded in the report that is issued. In many countries, the courts give instruction that the person will be examined even by force in cases that are threatening to society or that involve a public crime. With existence of a crime that is like an epidemic or that harms society, examination of the person may be carried without consent. Thus, with an emergency case, or if the person may die if not treated, examining the person and treating without consent will not conflict with ethical principles (American Academy of Psychiatry and the Law; Niveau and Welle 2018; Völlm et al. 2018; Taborda and Arboleda-Flórez 2006). In cases of hunger strike or death fasting, the application of medical treatment to people without their consent has been discussed (Taborda and Arboleda-Flórez 2006; Robertson 2000). The treatment decision of these people is left to the physicians (the Declaration of Malta-Marbella).

In case the person rejects a forensic psychiatric examination, what is said may not be relied upon. It is also probable that the person does not talk at all in the interview. It should be considered that many people may have been deceptive in a forensic examination as well. In the interview, the facial expression of the patient should be followed. In the diagnosis of many diseases, tests help in the verification of the diagnosis by providing objective data. The existence of a personality disorder in a patient, a lack of cooperation with the physician while providing an anamnesis, nonconformity with the disease or a case with information provided in detail should be examined carefully as to deception. For forensic patients, because the person could possess an advantage from the report obtained from the examination, care should be taken of deception, but the patient should not be directly approached as such (Turan Yurtsever N 2019). For forensic patients, if no decision may be taken based on an examination, the patient should be hospitalized and should be kept track of by obtaining the opinion of other members of the profession. The physician should attach findings that support his opinion with the video recording of the interview or in the outcome section of the report that is issued. The final decision should be made by the judge or prosecutor (Robertson 2000).

Liability of Confidentiality

The physician bears the task to maintain the personal privacy of his psychiatric patient, as with every patient. But with forensic cases, the physician bears a liability that lies between the legal order and ethics, which could be conflicting in the aspect of declaration (American Academy of Psychiatry and the Law; Niveau and Welle 2018; Taborda and Arboleda-Flórez 2006; Robertson 2000). The physician should resolve this with his patient before the interview. Firstly, he should ask the patient why he came and why he is there, meaning that he is questioning the level of consciousness of the patient and the existence of a forensic case, and therefore he grasps whether he accepts being examined. If the patient knows the reason for the examination and possesses legal capacity, the subsequent phase is the informed consent and the liability of confidentiality that is the responsibility of the physician in clinical interviews. However, the forensic patient should be informed of the fact that this interview will not be between physician and patient, but that the information that the patient gives may be shared with the legal authorities upon the request of the court (Arboleda-Florez 2006; Simon and Gold 2010).

Procurement of the environment for the examination where patients will share their private information is the task of the psychiatrist. If the telephone is continuously ringing during the interview or examination or someone enters the room, this affects the quality of the examination. The presence of other people in the environment is not desirable for focusing on the interview, both from the aspect of the physician and the patient, and in order that the information that is shared remains private. The information that the patient has given should be taken down as notes as told by the person without being changed. The physician should keep the details of the information that he received from his patient in a way to hinder access by others to his personal notes. He should submit the information relating to the patient electronically or as a hospital report in a way to ensure that they are comprehensible to colleagues, but without details (Cetin 2019). If he shares the relevant details, it is appropriate that he transmits them in a sealed envelope by a safe courier. In conformity with the rules of ethics of the Psychiatry Association of Turkey, with the purpose of protection and improving the mental health of the patient, it may be shared with relatives as far as necessary with consent of the patient, or it may be shared with another specialist for the purpose of consulting (Cetin 2019)). The physician may not share the private information of his patient with others on personal, occupational, academic, political, administrative or medical grounds without his consent. At the same time, the psychiatrist may not obtain information from others without the consent of the patient (Cetin 2019).

Even if the liability of maintaining the secrecy of the patient is a significant ethical principle, in forensic cases where it is harmful for the patient or others, or it poses a threat to another's life, these are exceptional cases in which this ethical principle may be disrupted. There are differing opinions among psychiatrists and even among physicians around the world in this matter (Appelbaum, 1997, Fox and Levy 2013, Robertson 2000).

Case 2

A patient of Dr. Mehmet with obsessive complaints was late for the 2nd check-up appointment. The patient relates that he washes his hands many times when leaving his house despite medication treatment. He leaves the house with difficulty due to checking lamps and taps many times. He returns to the house two times in order to check whether he had locked the door. Dr. Mehmet realizes that his patient trusted him compared to previous interviews and he continues with the interview in order to detail the past history of the patient. The patient relates that in the past he was involved with a crime at the starting period of his disease. He often dreamt of this event and even he woke up many times to wash his hands. When Dr. Mehmet asked about the type of incident that his patient went through and what kind of things he dreamt of, the patient relates that while he was sitting in the park with his closest friend at night at a young age, a man came over to them and swore at him. When he asked for an improper relationship, he and his friend got angry at this man and beat him up. But, after a while, the man did not move and when they realized that he had died, they escaped from the place and they did not talk about this ever again. He relates that he subsequently dreamt of the man and became angry at him, and dirtied himself all over his body. He then was relieved after he washed his hands many times. Dr. Mehmet gathered very significant information from his patient in his diagnosis and at the same time, grasped information relating to a serious case of crime that happened in the past. It is easy to diagnose and treat the patient from this point on. However, what should the doctor do with the information at hand?

In some cases, the psychiatrist may obtain criminal information while receiving the story of his patient. If the matter that has been learned may give harm to the life of the patient or the lives of others, a case that happened in the past and that could give harm to the life of others, the advantage of the patient or the benefit to society will dominate over the privacy or the liability of confidentiality that belongs to the physician and it is required that this information be shared with the judicial authorities (Niveau and Welle 2018; Cetin 2019).

If the patient is inadequate for autonomous decision making with regard to providing accurate information due to his mental health or inadequate mental capacity, in this case the obligation to obtain information from his relatives arises for the advantage of the related person. However, the ability of people from whom information will be received to provide information relating to the patient as well as their nearness should be evaluated. If it will be received from people who are in a personal conflict with the patient and/or who possess advantage by reason of his disease, the physician should be careful with the information. Likewise, it is preferred to not receive information from people when it may give rise to improper situations for the patient in the future, for instance, school friends or colleagues of the patient (Cetin 2019; Simon and Gold 2010).

Impartiality, Justice

According to the Declaration of the World Medical Association, the physician is obliged to apply proper treatment for the best advantage of his patient without discriminating. However, it is well known that those arrested or convicts are subject to discrimination or bias far more when compared to others in society (Robertson 2000). Forensic psychiatrists should be impartial and show equal treatment without empathy to those arrested and without considering what offense they perpetrated in order to apply justice (Niveau and Welle 2018; Völlm et al. 2018, Robertson 2000). An objective examination should be carried out without being empathized with the statement of the victim. The same standard diagnosis and treatment should be applied as with similar patients (American Academy of Psychiatry and the Law).

As far as serious crimes are concerned, indignation may arise in society causing political pressure upon the forensic psychiatrist upon announcement in the media. An image that patients have been stigmatized by society and have no worth may arise. In many countries, the expert is evaluated in the same position as a court jury or prosecutor and they are expected to act as impartially and neutral as at the time of evaluating the situation (Arboleda-Florez 2006; Völlm et al. 2018).

Therefore, before accepting a case, a psychiatrist should reject being an expert if it will disrupt his neutrality. In general, such cases are indicated when the patient is a relative of the expert or if there is personal communication or a case of advantage for any reason (Appelbaum1997, American Academy of Psychiatry and the Law; Taborda and Arboleda-Flórez 2006).

If a mental disorder is present in a forensic case, and such people are hospitalized by force or are subject to legal procedures in the form of suspension from society, or are released into society based on the physician's report without being punished due to their mental disorders, the ethical correctness should be put to discussion (Calcedo 2006; Völlm et al. 2018; Robertson 2000).

The ability to make a decision about themselves and free will belonging to the persons should be respected. However, such freedoms may be restricted as part of temporary precautions in case of damage and hazard that such people pose to others (American Academy of Psychiatry and the Law; Calcedo 2006).

According to what is stated in the Declaration of the World Medical Association, the physician should firstly think about the advantage of his patient. However, cases in which the person may give harm to himself or others are excluded. Likewise, in many justice systems of countries, if the physician encounters a crime, he should make it known to the judicial authorities. On the other hand, as part of discussions, it is advised that the psychiatrist puts ethical declarations under protection despite legal coercion (Robertson 2000; Cetin 2019; Calcedo 2006). However, when crimes such as sexual assault, murder or child abuse are perpetrated against humanity and are being hidden, or when the perpetrators are protected or hidden, this does not coincide with the ethical principles (American Academy of Psychiatry and the Law).

Since the physician has access to details of the clinical information, he grasps the relevant facts relating to the forensic case (without incurring change), he becomes cognizant of what the legal application will be and what kind of clinical information the judicial authorities will need (Cetin 2019; Taborda and Arboleda-Flórez 2006). Some prosecutors or judges do not wish to provide the forensic documentation of a person to be examined by a physician. They expect that the physician issues a report solely based on the medical documentation and examination. However, being cognizant of the details of the forensic case at the time of the examination and replying to questions that respond to the need of the court are beneficial in hindering the patient from directing the physician, as well as the deception of patients in suspicious cases. No experienced physician will issue a report taking into consideration the forensic information. However, by comparing the forensic information and the clinical findings that relate to the patient, he issues a more objective and impartial report.

From the physician who treats a person, information that consists of objective findings may be requested. However, from the physician that applies the treatment, the issuance of a forensic psychiatric examination report should not be requested. This is necessary both from the aspect of not disrupting the neutrality of the physician who has built empathy at the time of the treatment and from the aspect of not disrupting the patient-physician relationship that will continue thereafter (American Academy of Psychiatry and the Law; Völlm et al. 2018).

It is not an approved approach that the physician that issue reports in the case of forensic cases ask for a fee for this action from the patients. According to the author, ensuring that the fee that the expert person will receive for the work that he did is fixed on an institutional basis, considering some specific standards, is necessary both from the aspect of the report and to hinder improper claims that may arise subsequently for the expert (Appelbaum1997; Fox and Levy 2013).

Case 3

A male patient age 43 who was under a physician's care by reason of a psychosis for 5 years works in a bank. However, he says that he has an attraction towards a woman age 25 who works at the same bank. He has been sending unnamed love letters to the woman for years. One month ago, as part of a control examination, he confessed that he obtained information that the woman was flirting with another man and he started to keep track of the woman. After the interview, he did not come for the control examination with the psychiatrist and did not respond to his calls. The psychiatrist says that he lost contact for follow-up and treatment of his patient and more importantly, he is anxious that his patient may cause a hazardous situation for the girl and boyfriend with whom he is obsessively in love. What kind of precautions should this psychiatrist take in terms of the patient and his relatives?

It is not probable that the psychiatrist should make known the matter as a crime to the judicial authorities to determine whether a crime exists, how the crime will be kept track of and whether there is a victimized suspect. However, to keep track of the hazard of the patient, the possibility that he will get involved in a crime, whether he is in a safe position for himself and others, and whether he carries on with his treatment is under the responsibility of the psychiatrist (Cetin 2019). In some situations, the psychiatrist himself may be at risk since he obtained private information from his patient (Simon and Gold 2010). If the level of hazard of his patient has increased, the psychiatrist may ask for consultation from his colleagues and may follow the path of making a joint decision and a joint announcement (Völlm et al. 2018).

Treatment

The psychiatrist may encounter such issues on an ethical basis at the time of treating a patient as a forensic case in a state of emergency (American Academy of Psychiatry and the Law): Whether the anamnesis provided by the patient had been correct or not; his state of autonomy and freedom has been disrupted since the patient was restricted legally; and increased security measures because of the risk of him committing suicide or escaping, etc. (Völlm et al. 2018). In the meantime, due to the triangle of patient-physician-prosecutor, the trust of the patient towards the physician has impaired and subsequently he does not establish adequate cooperation with the physician.

Case 4

Mrs. Suzan was a bipolar manic-depressive patient for the last 20 years and has two daughters aged 22 and 18. She rejects going to a therapist and taking her medication in recent months. She gets out of her bed barely for the lavatory and eats only a little of the food that has been provided. She continuously says that the world is a bad place, there is no place in which they can survive any longer and she cannot stand it anymore. She is thinking about what will happen to her daughters. When her daughters call the therapist and tell about the case, the therapist says that the patient has to get treated because of the thoughts of suicide and major depression and has to be brought to the hospital in some way, but the patient rejects this.

Capacity assessment is needed for abilities regarding a specific situation such as medical care decision. People should only be declared incapable when it has been firmly established that they are unable to make decisions or that they pose a serious risk for themselves and those around them because of their incapacity. This might require consultation with a therapist.

Psychiatrists should ensure that their service has strong links with general practitioners and their teams so that people with mental health problems can easily access appropriate levels of treatment and support (Royal College of Psychiatrists 2000).

CONCLUSION

The forensic psychiatrist has to evaluate his patient in conformity with occupational professionalism and without deviating from medical ethics codes. However, since each patient and the societal conditions in which they exist differ, the psychiatrist should be cognizant of the articles of law that apply in the region and should act in conformity with the concepts of autonomy, beneficence and justice when evaluating his patient.

REFERENCES

American Academy of Psychiatry & the Law Ethical Guidelines for the Practice of Forensic Psychiatry (2013). Retrieved from file:///C:/Users/UX310/Downloads/1990_Bookmatter_EthicalPracticeInPsychiatryAnd.pdf; Accessed in December, 14, 2020.

American Psychiatric Association (2020*). The Opinions of the Ethics Committee on the Principles of Medical Ethics.* Retrieved from file:///C:/Users/UX310/Downloads/Opinions-of-the-Ethics-Committee.pdf.

Appelbaum PS (1997). A Theory of Ethics for Forensic Psychiatry. *J Am Acad Psychiatry Law,* 25(3);233-247.

Arboleda-Florez J, (2006). Forensic psychiatry: contemporary scope, challenges and controversies. *World Psychiatry,* 5(2);87-91.

Calcedo A (2006). The ethical implications of forensic psychiatry practice. *World Psychiatry,* 5; 93-94.

Cetin B (2019). Ethics in Psychiatry In: *Contemporary Clinical Ethics* by Demirhan Erdemir A. and et al. Istanbul: Nobel Medical Publishing, 235-249.

Declaration of Malta-Marbella (1991). *World Medical Assembley.* Retrieved from https://elearning.icrc.org/detention/en/story_content/external_files/Malta%20Declaration.pdf.

Declaration of Tokyo (1975). *World Medical Association.* Retrieved from https://www.wma.net/what-we-do/medical-ethics/declaration-of-tokyo/.

Eastman N et al. (2018). *Handbook of Forensic Psychiatry Practices in Capital Cases.* London: Oxford Unversity Press.

Fox MI and Levy MI (2013). The Use of Forensic Psychiatry in Catastrophic Injury and Multi-Party Litigation. *BNA Insights*, 13 (23); 623-629.

Gelder M and et al. (2006). *Shorter Oxford Textbook of Psychiatry.* New York: Oxford University Press.

Igoumenou A (2020). *Ethical Issues in Clinical Forensic Psychiatry.* London: Springer.

Maier M (1994). Forensic Psychiatry: Clinical, Legal and Ethical Issues. *J Neurol Neurosurg Psychiatry,* 58;127.

Niveau G and Welle I (2018). Forensic psychiatry, one subspecialty with two ethics? A systematic review. *BMC Medical Ethics,* 19:25 doi.org/10.1186/s12910-018-0266-5.

Robert IS and Liza HG (2010). *The Textbook of Forensic Psychiatry.* Washington: American Psychiatric Publishing.

Robertson M (2000). *An Introduction to Psychiatric Ethics.* Syndney: Health Education & Training Institute.

Royal College of Psychiatrists (2000). *Good Psychiatric Practice Code of Ethics.* Retrieved from www.rcpsych.ac.uk (accessed in December, 01,2020).

Sen P et al. (2007). Ethical dilemmas in forensic psychiatry: Two illustrative cases. *J Med Ethics,* 33; 337-341.

Simon IR and Gold LM (2010). *Textbook of Forensic Psychiatry* (Second Edition). London: The American Psychiatric Publishing.

Taborda JGV, Arboleda-Flórez J (2006). Forensic psychiatry ethics: expert and clinical practices and research on prisoners. *Rev Bras Psiquiatr,* 28; 86-92.

The General Medical Council Practice Rules (2004) Retrieved from https://www.legislation.gov.uk/uksi/2004/2608/schedule/made (accessed in December, 11, 2020).

The World Medical Association. *The European Committee for the Prevention of Torture and Inhuman or Degrading Treatment or Punishment* (2017). https://www.coe.int/en/web/cpt/ home.

Turan Yurtsever N (2019). Forensic Psychiatry In: *Current Studies of Health Sciences I* by Ozgunen T. Ankara: Akademisyen Publishing. 41-62.

Völlm BA et al. (2018). European Psychiatric Association (EPA) guidance on forensic psychiatry: Evidence based assessment and treatment of mentally disordered offenders. *Europen Psychiatry,* 51; 58-73.

In: Forensic Psychiatry …
Editor: Nursen Turan Yurtsever
ISBN: 978-1-53619-530-9

Chapter 2

Criminal Responsibility and Legal Capacity

Abdulkadir Tabo[1,*] and Nursen Turan Yurtsever[2]
[1]The Council of Forensic Medicine, Turkey
[2] Forensic Medicine Department,
Marmara University, School of Medicine, Istanbul, Turkey

Abstract

Determining whether a person has legal capacity and criminal responsibility is the main task of forensic psychiatry. In order for a person to have legal capacity and/or criminal responsibility, they must be able to understand their actions. Mental illnesses and young age are factors that affect both legal capacity and criminal responsibility. The insanity defense is based on the principle that a person who cannot appreciate the nature of the crime due to a mental illness they had when they committed the crime, cannot distinguish right from wrong and therefore is not legally responsible for the crime. Schizophrenia and similar psychoses and affective disorders are the leading mental disorders affecting both criminal responsibility and legal capacity. In the evaluation of criminal responsibility in children, it is important to determine the minimum legal age for criminal responsibility

[*] Corresponding Author's E-mail: akadirtabo@yahoo.com.

and to take biopsychosocial development factors into account. In a forensic mental assessment, not only is the psychiatric history and mental disorders evaluated, but also a mental status examination, including attention, mood, thinking (form and structure), memory and cognitive function, is made. A basic approach to assessment of mental state of a person in accordance with medical ethics is discussed in this chapter.

CRIMINAL RESPONSIBILITY

Introduction

Modern criminal law is based on the belief that people are morally responsible beings and should not hurt others. Three factors are required in order for an action to be considered a crime: mens rea, actus reus and foreseeable punishment in law (Blau et al. 1993). The concepts of mens rea and actus reus are the basic elements of criminal responsibility. Actus reus, or guilty act, refers to conduct constituting an element of a crime. Mens rea, the guilty mind, refers to the intention to act or the state of mental health. Therefore, it is not enough for a person just to perform a criminal act; they have to be mentally responsible for it (Feuerstein et al. 2005; Math et al. 2015; Oncu and Sercan 2018). Psychiatric disorders and young age are conditions that affect criminal responsibility.

Insanity defenses are fundamentally a subject of criminal cases. They are based on the claim that the accused suffered from severe mental illness at the time of the crime, therefore could not recognize the nature of the crime, did not know right from wrong, and therefore is not legally responsible for the crime (Morse and Bonnie 2013; Math et al. 2015). Although the legal standards for insanity defenses vary from one country to another and from state to state, within the U.S., the basic concept that a state of disorder/inadequacy in mental function can affect the degree of responsibility for a crime is widely accepted (Morse and Bonnie 2013).

Forensic psychiatric evaluation aims at determining whether a person had a psychiatric disorder at the time of the crime that affects criminal responsibility. In terms of criminal responsibility, it is not enough for a person to be suffering from a mental disorder. It is essential to determine its temporal relationship with the crime. The insanity defense is not a medical concept but a legal one. Although forensic psychiatric opinions are taken into account, throughout the world the decision to accept or reject the defense is at the discretion of the courts (Math et al. 2015; Oncu and Sercan 2018).

The concept of criminal responsibility in patients with mental disorders has a long and complex history. In this sense, the case of Daniel M'Naghten (or McNaughtan) was a turning point in the history of forensic psychiatry. M'Naghten, who was mentally ill, attempted to assassinate the Prime Minister of England in 1843. His defense was bases on the theses put forward by the American psychiatrist Isaac Ray on the legal status of mental illness. As a result of this defense, M'Naghten was hospitalized instead of punished (Dalby 2006; Kelly 2009). This decision caused controversy and, over time, judges developed various "M'Naghten rules" with regards to the criminal responsibility of mentally ill patients (Dalby 2006; Allnutt et al. 2007). M'Naghten rules state that if the defendant who committed the crime is ill to a degree and severity that they cannot understand the nature and consequences of their actions at the time of the crime, they cannot be punished for them (Allnutt et al. 2007). M'Naghten rules have been applied in many countries, primarily the USA and England (Kelly 2009). These rules have been regarded as strict, looking for precise links between crime and illness or severe cognitive losses.

In 1962, the American Law Institute (ALI), added the basic capacity and assessment ability of the person as elements of criminal responsibility, in addition to the M'Naghten rules requirements (Selh et al. 2005; Sosyal 2012; AALP 2014; Oncu and Sercan 2018). In 1982, John Hinckley attacked US President Ronald Reagan. The court's decision holding that Hinckley was not guilty by reason of insanity caused intense public reaction (Slater and Hans 1984; Selh et al. 2005; AALP 2014; Oncu and Sercan 2018). As a result, the "Federal Insanity Defense Reform Act of 1984" was enacted. This law is generally considered to be a return to the historical rule of "distinguishing right from wrong" from the more flexible Durham rule (Seth et al. 2005; AALP 2014). According to this law, in order to avoid criminal responsibility, a person must be incapable of evaluating the wrongness or nature of their behavior, as a result of a mental illness or weakness (Oncu and Sercan 2018). Following the Hinckley incident, some U.S. states abolished the insanity defense in favor of a "guilty but mentally ill" approach (Melville and Naimark 2002; Melamed 2010). The problems posed by the removal or restriction of insanity defenses in people with criminal psychiatric illnesses have been criticized (Melamed 2010: Morse and Bonnie 2013).

Mental Illnesses and Crime

Throughout history, it has been thought that there is a relationship between violent behavior and mental illnesses. In early studies, it was reported that people with mental illnesses displayed less violent behavior compared to the rest of the society. However, later studies found that the crime rate among these patients was equal to or higher than society in general. This difference between studies may be related to the change in mental health policies after 1960, which and tended to treat patients more within the community (Rueve and Welton 2008; İnan S et al. 2018).

In recent years, an increasing number of studies have found that violence and criminal behavior are higher in people with mental disorders than in the general population. Yet, studies also show that, contrary to popular belief, most patients with mental disorders do not commit crimes, and mental disorders are responsible for a small fraction of all crimes (Fazel and Grann 2006). In some studies, it was found that while people with mental disorders are in general no more dangerous than the general population, there is a high-risk subgroup of patients, associated with previous criminal history, alcohol-substance abuse and non-adherence to treatment (Rueve and Welton 2008; Yee et al. 2011; İnan S et al. 2018).

Compared to the general population, the risk of violence is increased in cases of traumatic brain injury (Fazel et al. 2011), personality disorders (Yu et al. 2012), mental retardation (Hodgins 1992), and depression (Wallece et al. 1998; Arseneault et al. 2000). The rate of violence seen in substance abuse (Fazel et al. 2009) and antisocial personality disorder (Yu et al. 2012) is higher than in most psychiatric disorders (Swanson et al. 2015).

Schizophrenia and Similar Psychoses

Schizophrenia and similar psychoses and affective disorders are the leading mental disorders affecting criminal responsibility. The term psychosis is used to describe situations in which the ability to evaluate reality is lost. Schizophrenia, a psychotic disorder, is an illness in which symptoms such as delusions, hallucinations, disorganized behavior, avolition and apathy are seen (Sadock and Sadock 2007). Paranoid schizophrenia and substance abuse comorbidity have been found to be associated with an increased risk of violence (Richard-Devantoy et al. 2009).

There is a close relationship between psychotic symptoms and acts of violence (Krakowski et al. 1999). Violent behavior can be seen as part of disorganized or agitated behavior. Severe paranoid delusions, and especially auditory command hallucinations, can also lead to increased aggression. Violence increases with active psychotic symptoms and substance abuse, and most people had active psychotic symptoms while committing a crime (Junginger 1995; Junginger 1996; Krakowski et al. 1999; Appelbaum et al. 2000; Ural et al. 2013; Volovka 2013; Cinik et al. 2015). In first episode psychoses without prior treatment, the risk of homicide was found to be 15 times higher compared to that after treatment (Nielssen and Large 2010; Yee et al. 2011). The presence of comorbidities, such as young age, male gender, being in the acute phase of the disease, previous suicide attempt, non-compliance with treatment, past history of violence, substance abuse and antisocial personality disorder increase the risk of violence in schizophrenia (Volavka and Swanson 2010; Yee et al. 2011; Cinik et al. 2015). In a meta-analysis and review study, schizophrenia and other psychoses were found to be associated with violent crimes, particularly murder. (Fazel S et al. 2009). However, the risk of violence is not an issue for most schizophrenics and is associated with a small subgroup (Richard-Devantoy et al. 2009).

Affective Disorders

Studies investigating the relationship between bipolar disorder and violent behavior are relatively few. In a German study conducted on a large (n = 1561) group of affective disorder patients, the prevalence of violent behavior and crime of violence within 7 to 12 years after discharge was examined. The highest rate of violent behaviors and crimes of violence was observed in the manic disorder group. Violence and crime are extremely rare in those with major depressive disorder. It was determined that men were sixtimes more likely to commit crimes of violence than were women, for whom the most common crimes were embezzlement, theft and fraud; only one person in the study committed murder (Graz et al. 2009).

In a study conducted in the U.S. where National Comorbidity Survey data were evaluated, the lifetime aggressive behavior rate (as recorded in police or court records) was 12.2% for bipolar disorder and 1.9% for those without a mental illness. (Corrigan and Watson 2005; Volavka 2013). Alcohol/substance addiction, and paranoid and antisocial personality disorder comorbidity rates, are significantly higher in bipolar disorder and this increases the risk of violence (Grant et al. 2005; Latalova 2009).

Clinical observations show that the risk of violence is high during acute manic episodes (Binder and McNiel 1988; Barlow et al. 2000; Ballester et al. 2012). It has been reported that the symptom profile in mania (grandiose, impulsivity, impaired reasoning, lack of insight, psychotic symptoms) can increase the risk of committing offenses by predisposing the person to aggressive behavior (Quanbeck et al. 2004).

Some researchers have stated that the correlation between depression and violence is much more common than general believed (Rosenbaum and Bennett 1986; Malmquist 1995). In a study conducted among criminals sent for compulsory psychiatric treatment over a 22-year period, a diagnosis of bipolar disorder was found in 219 people, and the total crime rate was found to be higher in manic episodes than in depressive episodes. However, homicide rates were higher in depressive episodes, and homicide victims of patients in depressive episodes were more likely to be family members. While murder with altruistic motivation was higher in depressive episodes, impulsivity was found more common in manic episodes (Yoon J-H et al.

2012). Sometimes, in severe depressions with psychotic features, the patient may kill one or more of his family members with the delusion that he is rescuing them from a very tragic situation (altruistic homicide). Suicide after murder is common (Richard-Dvantoy S et al. 2008; Fovet et al. 2015).

Case 1

Mrs. M is 28 years old. She is an elementary school graduate and has been married for eight years. Her husband is a manual laborer. She has one son; a year ago, she killed her younger son under difficult circumstances. She has been sent by the court for a mental health assessment, to determine whether she has criminal responsibility regarding the death. In her history, Mrs. M stated that her mental problems started before she fell pregnant with her second child; after a psychiatric evaluation she diagnosed with major depression and placed on anti-depressants; her complaints were alleviated by the medication and she had an unplanned pregnancy. Her doctor stopped the medication due to her pregnancy, but she started taking the antidepressants again after the sixth month of her pregnancy as her complaints were aggravated. After the delivery; her depressive complaints were aggravated: She complained of low mood, not being able to enjoy life, lethargy, loss of appetite, sleeplessness, not taking care of or feeding her baby, and feeling inadequate as a mother. Her doctor recommended hospitalization but she refused and she was started on a new anti-depressant. This new medication did not help and her complaints became worse approximately four months after her delivery. She also stated that she never held her baby and that it was her mother who usually looked after the baby; she could not stand the baby's crying; she did not feel any love towards the baby; she saw him as the reason for her problems; and she thought that life was empty and meaningless because of him. One day, when her mother went out to the supermarket and left her alone with the baby, he started crying. She said she did not know what to do; she could not stand the sound of his crying, so she pushed a pillow over his face and the crying stopped; she saw that the baby was not breathing anymore; she went into her own room and laid down; and she was woken up by her mother's screams when she returned from the supermarket. She was hospitalized in a psychiatric hospital for about six weeks immediately after the incident and was diagnosed with postpartum depression; she still continued to take medication, which alleviated her complaints; she felt very sad and guilty because of the death of her baby even though doctors associated this incident with her disease; she did not have any mental problems during her first pregnancy or after her first delivery; she did not use alcohol or any substance; she had no criminal history before the incident; she had a good relationship with her child now; her husband and family supported her after the incident. She describes affective disorder history in her family.

During the psychiatric examination, it was observed that she cried from time to time and had a depressive affect while describing the event. There was no thought or perception disorder. Her thoughts of guilt about the child she killed were evident in thought contents. She described a slight decrease in her social and professional functionality. As a result of the examination of her psychiatric history, psychiatric examination, medical records before and after the incident, and forensic documents related to the incident, no psychiatric illness that would affect her criminal responsibility was detected. However, it was decided that there was no criminal responsibility for the crime due to "postpartum depression," as such was understood at the time of the crime.

Criminal Responsibility in Children

Juvenile delinquency is a serious, worldwide problem (Pardini 2016). The age at which a child's criminal responsibility begins is important in terms of protection of children's rights. The age of onset of criminal responsibility varies from 7 to 18 years (Erdener 2015; Pillay and Willows 2015). Upon achieving the age of criminal responsibility, a child or adolescent is considered to have the same capacity as an adult in understanding the purpose, seriousness and possible consequences of a crime (Noroozi et al. 2018).

The assessment of criminal responsibility in children is a complex issue. Some international standards and principles have been established, but these are very general and cannot provide complete solutions in specific cases (Pillay and Willows 2015). In the forensic psychiatric process, each case must be evaluated individually. When evaluating juvenile delinquency, it is important to take biopsychosocial factors into account (Erdener 2015).

Factors that Affect Criminal Responsibility in Children

Childhood and adolescence are the periods in which personality begins to take shape and the socialization process is most intense. Besides the individual characteristics of the child, family and socioeconomic factors also affect the child's socialization process. In this process, the child's tendency towards crime may emerge (Williams-Evans and Myers 2004; Savolainen et al. 2018). In evaluating the criminal responsibility of children, neuroanatomical developments, neurochemical changes and psychosocial factors that occur in the brain during adolescence should be taken into account (Barbalat et al. 2010; Burke 2011; Erdener 2015; Yıldız 2018).

The extent of development of adolescents' decision-making and judgment capacities is important in determining their criminal responsibilities. Compared to adults, adolescentshave inadequate judgmental and decision-making capacities, which may reduce their responsibility for criminal acts (Yıldız 2018). Psychosocial factors and the immaturity of the neural systems in the brain that regulate risk-taking-seeking and impulsivity can negatively affect their decision-making abilities and thus their criminal responsibility (Llamas and Marinaro 2020).

Decision making is a complex and multidimensional process. Reasoning and judgment together affect the decision-making process. Reasoning describes the cognitive capacity required to process information. Judgment, on the other hand, is the ability to make a connection between many possible consequences of decisions and their degrees of significance (Kambam & Thompson 2009; Yıldız 2018). Along with cognitive capacity, psychosocial maturation also plays an important role in the decision-making process. Adolescents' psychosocial immaturity can lead to criminal behavior by negatively affecting the judgment and decision-making processes (Kambam and Thompson 2009; Yıldız 2018). Mature decision-making ability is not sufficiently developed until early adulthood (Halpern-Felsher and Cauffman 2001; Archer et al. 2012; Yıldız 2018). In the decision-making process, adolescents also differ from adults in terms of time perception and future orientation, and focus more on short-term results. They prefer to make sudden decisions rather than rational decisions. While calculating profit and loss against risk, they focus more on short-term and positive results of decisions. They perceive risks at a lower level compared to adults. Adolescents are easily influenced by their peers and value their approval. Therefore, they make more risky decisions while in a group (Barbalat et al. 2010; Yıldız 2018).

Children's moral development strongly impacts their ability to evaluate the rightness or wrongness of their actions. Moral development requires both the ability to judge a crime in accordance with moral principles and to give appropriate emotional responses (such as guilt and empathy) to the crime. The age factor is very important for moral development. (Malti et al. 2010; Erdener 2015; Yıldız 2018). Moral reasoning capacity increases with age (Erdener 2015). In a comprehensive meta-analysis study, it was shown that there is a significant relationship between low moral judgment and juvenile delinquency, and children involved in crime have lower moral judgment capabilities (Stams et al. 2006; Yıldız 2018).

Impulsivity can lead to significant behavioral problems and criminality in adolescents. Impulsivity is defined as acting without adequately evaluating alternatives and "giving rapid and unplanned responses to internal and external stimuli by ignoring possible negative consequences on both oneself and others" (Moeller et al. 2001; Schreiber et al. 2012). Maturation of the frontal lobe plays a key role in the regulation of emotions, impulse control, the ability to judge consequences, and executive functions. Studies show that this maturation process continues until early adulthood (Alvarez and Emory 2006; Archer et al. 2012).

Studies report that children with criminal tendencies share certain psychosocial risk factors: Lack of emotional stability, being male, having low intelligence, a history of attention deficit and hyperactivity disorder, conduct disorder, alcohol or substance abuse, history of trauma, school adjustment problems, conflict between parents, broken family, and criminal social environment are each associated with juvenile delinquency (Erdener 2015; Taskiran et al. 2017; Savolainen et al. 2018).

Legal Capacity

Introduction

In the twentieth century, some important socio-demographic changes made legal capacity assessment more prominent. The world population is aging and so the cognitive and physical changes that are occurring in the aging population with loss of decision-making skills being prominent (Donnelly 2007; Scott 2008; Moye and Marson 2007; Marshall, Kapp 2010).

Legal capacity should in particular be assessed if the person's decision puts themselves, or others, at risk of harm or mistreatment because of its severe consequences. The possibility of mental illness and intellectual disability should also be assessed if the person's decision was very different from their usual decisions, conflicts with the person's usual preferences, or is different from the decision that most people would make in the same circumstances (Calcedo-Barba et al. 2020).

With a presumption of legal capacity, the expert should consider the balance between a person's right to make their own decisions and the extent to which that person's health or safety might be in danger if they cannot make an appropriate decision (Purser K., Rosenfeld T 2014). The rules that capacity is presumed and that persons with legal capacity are allowed to make decisions for themselves reflects society's strong ethical preference for maintaining the individual's decisional autonomy (Calcedo-Barba et al. Purser K., Rosenfeld T 2014). It is important to understand that if a person is not allowed to confront a difficult decision and its consequences, their right to be in control of their life is denied (Marshall, Kapp 2010).

Each individual has the right to take their own chances and make their own mistakes if legal capacity is not unsound. But mental capacity is not immutable and something easily measured. A person's mental capacity may depend on the type of decision being made, whether the decision is simple, and the person's familiarity with the subject matter. The person's level of education, intelligence and how the information is processed are all important factors influencing a person's ability to make a particular decision (Scott 2008Marshall, Kapp2010). It is well known that mental capacity can be regained when one is well and lost during periods of mental illness. In such cases, legal capacity should be reassessed when an important business or financial or similar weighty decision must be made (Scott 2008; Marshall, Kapp 2010).

A person with legal capacity has the right to make decisions for themselves and have an autonomous life, while someone lacking legal capacity requires a lawful authority or lawfully-appointed representative to make decisions on their behalf. For example, consent to a medical treatment will be invalid if it has been given by a person who does not have legal capacity, and treating such a person without consent may give rise to civil and/or criminal sanctions (Marshall, Kapp 2010).

Ethical Approaches to Assessment

Legal capacity assessment has important ethical, clinical and legal aspects. When carrying out a psychiatric assessment on a person whose mental capacity is uncertain, or who is accused of a crime, some key points should be kept in mind (Gelder M. et al. 2005; Scott 2008)

Prepare before the interview: Understand the purpose of the examination, obtain details of the crime, statements of witnesses and all reports about the person's social situation, and confirm (or refute) their accuracy during the interview.

Introduce yourself and then ask about his understand of his current circumstances. It is important to communicate to the person what you are doing, in order to get the person to participate willingly in the process. Record all comments in the person's own words.

Take a detailed history of any physical diseases.

Obtain a careful history of previous psychiatric disorders and treatments. Obtain further information from relatives and other relevant individuals

Determine his present mental state and intelligence level and request further investigation, as the case may require.

Assessment of legal capacity concerns not only the evaluation of psychiatric history and mental disorders, but also a mental status examination including attention, mood, thinking (form and structure), memory and cognitive functioning (Gelder M. et al. 2005; Purser K., Rosenfeld T 2014)).

A person with legal capacity is able to do all of the following (Moye and Marson 2007; Scott 2008):

Understand	Cognitively grasp and retain information
	Process information regarding available options and risks
	Understand relevant information
	Comprehend basic information about a problem and its possible solutions
	Predict the risks and benefits associated with possible solutions
Appreciate	Appreciate the situation and its possible consequences
	Recognize how a problem or solution pertains to one's own situation
Reason	Utilize logical thought processes in making a choice
Communicate	Render a clear choice

The person's level of education and intelligence, how the information is presented, the complexity of the situation, previous decisions and actions, and cultural or religious beliefs are all factors that influence a person's understanding, appreciation and communication abilities (Scott 2008; Purser, Rosenfeld 2014)). Communication ability is often preserved despite impairments in the other decision- making abilities (Scott 2008). Before the person is assessed as lacking decision-making capacity, everything possible should be done to support them in making a decision (Scott 2008).

Psychometric inventories can provide useful, informative data that assists the clinician to come to an opinion regarding one or more elements of an individual's mental ability (Porser, Rosenfeld 2014). However, there is no psychometric inventory designed to measure legal capacity alone. General intellectual ability, memory and ability to learn, attention and concentration, verbal comprehension and expression, reasoning, information processing and executive functioning can be assessed by tests. Consideration should also be given to the use of appropriate tests when using psychometric assessment inventories (Purser, Rosenfeld 2014; Marshall, Kapp 2010).

The neurologic and neuropsychological criteria that indicate a possible inadequacy in the clinical description of mental adequacy have been classified in the forms of attention, memory, speech, perception, deduction, and description of emotions(Can et al. 2006; Turan Yurtsever N 2019)). When making an evaluation of someone's legal capacity, there is a clear need to apply multidisciplinary examination including neurologic and psychiatric examination, to explore the person's adjustment to the daily life and to find whether he has a connection with judicial or criminal cases (Porser, Rosenfeld 2014; Turan Yurtsever 2019)).

If the court needs to know whether a person possessed legal capacity on a prior date, it would be highly relevant to have an examination report that pertains to the relevant date that was issued by a mental health specialist. However, such reports often do not exist. In such cases, whatever medical documentation (e.g., medical examinations, reports, prescriptions) that is nearest to the relevant date should be obtained. In addition, statements by relatives and witnesses that explain the actions taken on the relevant date, as well as information regarding the attitudes and behaviors of the person on, before and after the relevant date, the criminal state of the person, his personality, and the connections between the behavior and the benefit to the person concerned, should all be gathered from the judicial inquiry file (Porser, Rosenfeld 2014; Marshall, Kapp 2010; Turan Yurtsever 2019).

The outcome of a legal capacity assessment should always be documented, as it is critical for clinicians to evidence how they came to a conclusion that a person has, or lacks, decision-making capacity (Marshall, Kapp 2010). The forensic psychiatrist should be aware that the court will see the report, and the report should be written in a way that is understandable by judges, lawyers and juries at court (Gelder M et al. 2005).

A court report should contain following material:

1. The psychiatrist's full name, qualifications, and present appointment.
2. Information about the subject, such as full name, age, gender, communication ability.
3. Sources of information, including documents that have been examined.
4. Family and personal history of the subject; usually this need not be given in great detail. The focus should be on information relevant to the diagnosis and disposition.
5. A summary of the questions asked and answers given.
6. Documentation of the assessment process.
7. Present mental state of the subject. A detailed mental assessment and a general diagnosis should be given in the terms of the relevant mental health act (mental illness, mental impairment, or psychopathic disorder).
8. Mental state of the subject at the time of the relevant events
9. Conclusions (Gelder M et al. 2005; Scott 2008)

The report must state whether the subject currently has legal capacity, and his future prospects (Marshall, Kapp2010; Scott 2008). In particularly, in the case of bipolar affective disorders, it should be stated in the report that the subject might heal and be able to act based on his free will, since in the case of temporary mental disorders the court may terminate the custodianship (Balcioglu and Baser, 2008).

Case 2

Ms. H. is a 40 years old woman, a university graduate, divorced, having a son at the age of 10. In order to determine whether she has a psychiatric disease, which would hinder her from obtaining custody of her son, she has been referred by the court for a legal capacity assessment. She says that she divorced her spouse almost six years ago because he cheated on her; Her son was nine at the time of the divorce, and thereafter spent weekends with his father in conformity with the court verdict. Almost 6 months after the divorce, her son, after spending the weekend with his father, stated that his butt hurt. Ms. H did not give the matter close attention, thinking that it might be a case of constipation. Eventually, she realized that the child was calmer after being with the father; when he occasionally complained about a pain in his butt, the thought occurred to her that her ex-spouse may have abused her son. She examined the boy while he was asleep, and detected a rash around his anus, which caused her to believe that this was a case of rape. When she had her son examined by a pediatric doctor, the doctor stated that this was not something abnormal; nevertheless she was not convinced. She took her son to be examined by other doctors, who reiterated that that was not a case of rape; however, the rash and pain continued, so she filed a complaint with the prosecutor. The child was then given a judicially-ordered examination, which again found no evidence of rape. She did not believe the finding and thought her spouse had wrongfully influenced the doctors by making use of his circles; when the child did not meet his father his complaints of rash and pain subsided, which was the proof that the incident had happened. She acknowledged that during her marriage her spouse was a very attentive father to his son; did not use alcohol and substances; and was well-liked in his circles; and to this day could not believe that he could have perpetrated such "a pervertedness." While the son had defended his father, saying that his father had not done anything bad, the child may not remember it since her spouse had raped him after giving him a sleeping pill; the child had been in a drowsy state every time after returning from his father; she now better understood what had happened. She said that she does not use alcohol and substances; is not receiving psychiatry treatment; had been examined before and was issued a mental disease diagnosis, which is not correct. She asserted that what she was saying is true; that she wishes to get the custody of her child; and that the child is living with her for the time being and she does not let him see his father.

The psychiatrist's conclusion was that Ms. H was having a discrete paranoid delusion, had not told any hallucinations; did not possess any insight and had distorted judgement. As such, "a paranoid disorder" was diagnosed. Based on an examination of the divorce lawsuit file, it became evident that she had been diagnosed with a "paranoid disorder" at the psychiatry hospital where she had previously been referred by the court. The court thus found no evidence of rape and, based on the evaluation of the child psychiatrist, it was determined that the child had no mental disorder and had truthfully denied the allegations of his mother. The decision was made that Ms. H did not possess legal capacity due to a paranoid disorder, and that it would not be appropriate for her to have custody of the child.

CONCLUSION

Decision making is a complex and multidimensional process. Reasoning and judgment together affect the decision-making process. Reasoning describes the cognitive capacity required to process information. Judgment, on the other hand, is the ability to make a connection between many possible consequences of decisions and their degree of significance. An assessment of legal capacity and criminal responsibility concerns not only the evaluation of psychiatric history and mental disorders, but also a mental status examination including attention, mood, thinking (form and structure), memory and cognitive function. In making this assessment, medical ethics principles should be practiced, including respecting a person's privacy and autonomy.

REFERENCES

American Academy of Psychiatry and the Law (AALP 2014). Practice guideline for forensic psychiatric evaluation of defendants raising the insanity defense. *J Am Acad Psychiatry Law*, *42*(4 suppl), 3-76. https://www.aapl.org/docs/pdf/Insanity Defense Guidelines.pdf. Accessed: 15 Nov 2020.

Allnutt, S., Samuels, A. & O'Driscoll, C. (2007). The insanity defence: from wild beasts to M'Naghten. *Australasian Psychiatry*, *15*(4), 292-8.

Alvarez, J. A. & Emory, E. (2006). Executive function and the frontal lobes: a meta-analytic review. *Neuropsychol Rev*, *16*, 17–42.

Appelbaum, P. S., Robbins, P. C. & Monahan, J. (2000). Violence and delusions: data from the Mac Arthur Violence Risk Assesment Study. *Am J Psychiatry*, *157*, 566-72.

Archer, T., Oscar-Berman, M., Blum, K. & Gold, M. (2012). Neurogenetics and epigenetics in impulsive behaviour: impact on reward circuitry. *J Genet Syndr Gene Ther*, *3*(3), 1000115.

Balcioglu, I. & Baser, S. Z. (2008). Problems of Doctors in Forensic Psychiatry During Practice. *Istanbul University Cerrahpasa Medical School Continous Education Activities*, *62*, 41-48.

Ballester, J., Goldstein, T., Goldstein, B., Obreja, M., Axelson., et al. (2012). Is bipolar disorder specifically associated with aggression? *Bipolar Disord*, *14*, 283-290.

Barbalat, G., Domenech, P., Vernet, M. & Fourneret, P. (2010). Risk-taking in adolescence: a neuroeconomics approach. Review. *Encephale*, *36*(2), 147-54.

Barlow, K., Grenyer, B. & Ilkiw-Lavalle, O. (2000). Prevalence and precipitants of aggression in psychiatric inpatient units. *Aust N Z J Psychiatry*, *34*, 967-974.

Binder, R. L. & McNiel, D. E. (1988). Effects of diagnosis and context on dangerousness. *Am J Psychiatry*, *145*, 728-732.

Blau, G. I., Mcginley, H. & Pasewark, R. (1993). Understandıng the use of the ınsanıty defense. *Journal of Clinical Psychology*, *49* (3), 435-40.

Burke, A. S. (2011). Under construction: Brain formation, culpability, and the criminal justice system. Review. *Int J Law Psychiatry*, *34*(6), 381-5.

Calcedo-Barba, A., Fructuoso, A., Martinez-Raga, J., Paz, S., Sanchez de Carmona, M. & Vicens, E. (2020). A meta-review of literatüre reviews assessing the capacity of patients with severe mental disorders to make decisions about their healthcare. *BMC Psychiatry*, *20*, 339.

Can, Y., Sercen, M., Saatcioglu, O., Soysal, H. & Uygun, N. (2006). Form of Legal Capacity Evaluation: Validity, Reliabililty and Sensibility (Hukuki Ehliyeti Değerlendirme Formu (HEDEF). Geçerlilik, Güvenilirlik ve Duyarlılık). *Cilinical Psychiatry*, *9*, 5-16.

Cinik, E., Guclu, O., Senormanci, O., Aydin, E., Erkiran, M. & Husnu, Erkmen. (2015). Substance use effects on the characteristics of crime and violence in schizophrenia. *Anatolian Journal of Psychiatry*, *16*, 104-12.

Corrigan, P. W. & Watson, A. C. (2005). Findings from the National Comorbidity Survey on the frequency of violent behavior in individuals with psychiatric disorders. *Psychiatry Res*, *136*, 153-162.

Dalby, J. T. (2006). "The case of Daniel McNaughton: Let's get the story straight". *American Journal of Forensic Psychiatry*, *27*, 17–32.

Donnelly, M. (2007). Assessing Legal Capacity: Process and the Operation of the Functional Test. *Judicial Studies Institute Journal January*, *2*, 141-68.

Erdener, E. (2015). Examination of the perception of the legal meaning and the consequences of crime among children and the socio-cultural factors influencing these perceptions with respect to criminal responsibility. *J For Med*, *29*(2), 92-111.

Fazel, S. & Grann, M. (2006). The population impact of severe mental illness on violent crime. *Am J Psychiatry*, *163*, 1397-403.

Fazel, S., Gulati, G., Linsell, L., Geddes, J. R. & Grann, M. (2009). Schizophrenia and violence: systematic review and meta-analysis. *PLoS Med*, *6*(8), e1000120.

Fazel, S., Lichtenstein, P., Grann, M. & Långström, N. (2011). Risk of violent crime in individuals with epilepsy and traumatic brain injury: a 35-year Swedish population study. *PLoS Med*, (8)*12*, e1001150.

Feuerstein, S., Fortunati, F., Morgan, C. A., Coric, V., Temporini, H. & Southwick, S. (2005). The insanity defense. *Psychiatry* (Edgmont), *2*(9), 24–25.

Fovet, T., Geoffroy, P. A., Vaiva, G., Adins, C., Thomas, P. & Amad, A. (2015). Individuals with bipolar disorder and their relationship with the criminal justice system: a critical review. *Psychiatric Services*, *66*, 348-53.

Gelder, M., Harrison, P. & Cowen, P. (2005). *Shorter Oxford Textbook of Psychiatry*. NewYork: Oxford University Press., 729-757.

Grant, B. F., Stinson, F. S., Hasin, D. S., Dawson, D. A., Chou, S. P., et al. (2005). Prevalence, correlates, and comorbidity of bipolar I disorder and axis I and II disorders: results from the National Epidemiologic Survey on Alcohol and Related Conditions. *J Clin Psychiatry*, *66*, 1205-15.

Graz, C., Etschel, E., Schoech, & Soyka, M. (2009). Criminal behaviour and violent crimes in former inpatients with affective disorder. *Journal of Affective Disorders*, *117*, 98–103.

Halpern-Felsher, B. L. & Cauffman, E. (2001). Costs and benefits of a decision: Decision-making competence in adolescents and adults. *Journal of Applied Developmental Psychology*, *22*(3), 257-73.

Hodgins, S. (1992). Mental disorder, intellectual deficiency, and crime. *Arch Gen Psychiatry*, *49*, 476-83.

İnan, S., Yildizhan, E. & Oncu, F. (2018). The disease history, sociodemographics, and criminal features of the homicidal forensic psychiatric patients. *Turk Psikiyatri Derg*, *29*(4), 258-68.

Jablensky, A. (2000). Epidemiology of schizophrenia: the global burden of disease and disability. *Eur Arch Psychiatr Clin Neurosc*, *250*, 274-28.

Junginger, J. (1995). Command hallucinations and the prediction of dangerousness. *Psychiatr Serv*, *46*, 911-14.

Junginger, J. (1996). Psychiosis and violence: the case for a content analysis of psychotic experience. *Schizophr Bull*, *22*, 91-103.

Kambam, P. & Thompson, C. (2009). The development of decision-making capacities in children and adolescents: psychological and neurological perspectives and their implications for juvenile defendants. *Behavioral Sciences and the Law*, *27*, 173–90.

Kelly, B. D. (2009). Criminal insanity in 19th-century Ireland, Europe and the United States: cases, contexts and controversies. *International Journal of Law and Psychiatry*, *32*, 362–368.

Knoll, J. L. & Resnick, P. J. (2008). Insanity defense evaluations: toward a model for evidence-based practice. *Brief Treat Crisis Interv*, *8*(1), 92-110.

Krakowski, M., Czobar, P. & Chou, J. C. (1999). Course of violence in patients with schizophrenia: relationship to clinical symptoms. *Schizophr Bull*, *25*(3), 505-17.

Lamberti, J. S. (2007). Understanding and preventing criminal recidivism among adults with psychotic disorders. *Psychiatr Serv*, *58*, 773-781.

Latalova, K. (2009). Bipolar disorder and aggression. *Int J Clin Pract*, *63*, 889-99.

Llamas, N. E. & Marinaro, J. Á. (2020). Neuroscience in youth criminal law: reconsidering the measure of punishment in Latin America. *Front Psycho* 11: 302. https:// www.ncbi.lm.nih.gov/pmc/articles/ PMC7052333/pdf/fpsyg-11-0302.pdf. Accessed: 20 Nov 2020.

Malmquist, C. P. (1995). Depression and homicidal violence. *Int. J. Law Psychiatry*, *18*, 145–162.

Malti, M., Gasser, L. & Gutzwiller-Helfenfinger, E. (2010). Children's interpretive understanding, moral judgments, and emotion attributions: relations to social behaviour. *Br J Dev Psychol*, *28*(2), 275-92.

Marshall, B. & Kapp, J. D. (2010). Legal Issues Arising in the Process of Determining Decisional Capacity in Older Persons. *Care Management Journals*, *11*(2), 101-107. DOI: 10.1891/1521-0987.11.2.101

Math, S. B., Kumar, C. N. & Moirangthe, S. (2015). Insanity defense: past, present, and future. *Indian J Psychol Med*, *37*(4), 381–87.

Melamed, Y. (2010). Mentally ill persons who commit crimes: punishment or treatment? *J Am Acad Psychiatry Law*, *38*, 100-3.

Melville, J. D. & Naimark, D. (2002). Punishing the insane: the verdict of guilty but mentally ill. *J Am Acad Psychiatry Law*, *30*, 553–5.

Morse, S. J. & Bonnie, R. J. (2013). Abolition of the insanity defense violates due process. *J Am Acad Psychiatry Law*, *41*, 488–95.

Moye, J. & Marson, D. C. (2007). Assessment of Decision-Making Capacity in Older Adults: An Emerging Area of Practice and Research. *Journal of Gerontology: Psychological Sciences*, *62*(1), P3-P11.

Mullen, P., Burgess, P., Wallace, C., Palmer, S. & Ruschena, D. (2000). Community care and criminal offending in schizophrenia. *Lancet*, *355*, 614 – 17.

Nielssen, O. & Large, M. (2010). Rates of homicide during the first episode of psychosis and after treatment: a systematic review and meta-analysis. *Schizophr Bull*, *36*, 702 – 12.

Noroozi, M., Singh, I. & Fazel, M. (2018). Evaluation of the minimum age for consent to mental health treatment with the minimum age of criminal responsibility in children and adolescents: a global comparison. *Evid Based Mental Health*, *21*(3), 82-86.

Oncu, F. & Sercan, M. (2018). *Ceza Hukukunda Adli Psikiyatri*. Editör: Uygur N. Adli Psikiyatri Uygulama Kılavuzu. pp. 33-66. Ankara: Türkiye Psikiyatri Derneği Yayınları (3.Baskı). [*Forensic Psychiatry in Criminal Law*]

Pardini, D. (2016). Empirically based strategies for preventing juvenile delinquency. *Child Adolesc Psychiatr Clin N Am*, *25*(2), 257-68.

Pillay, A. L. & Willows, C. (2015). Assessing the criminal capacity of children: a challenge to the capacity of mental health professionals. *J Child Adolesc Ment Health*, *27*(2), 91–101.

Purser, K. & Rosenfeld, T. (2014). Evaluation of legal capacity by doctors and lawyers: The need for collaborative Assessment. *Ethics and Law*, *201*(8), 483-485.

Quanbeck, C. D., Stone, D. C., Scott, C. L., McDermott, B. E., Altshuler, L. L. & Frye, M. A. (2004). Clinical and legal correlates of inmates with bipolar disorder at time of criminal arrest. *Journal of Clinical Psychiatry*, *65*, 198–203.

Richard-Devantoy, S., Chocard, A. S., Bouyer-Richard, A. I., Duflot, J. P., Lhuillier, J. P., et al. (2008). Homicide and psychosis: criminological particularities of schizophrenics, paranoiacs and melancholic. A review of 27 expertises. *Encephale*, *34*, 322-9.

Rosenbaum, M. & Bennett, B. (1986). Homicide and depression. *Am J Psychiatry*, *143*, 367–370.

Porser, J. K. & Rosenfeld, T. (2014). Evaluation of legal capacity by doctors and lawyers: the need for collaborative assessment. *The Medical journal of Australia*, *483*, 1-4.

Rueve, M. E. & Welton, R. S. (2008). Violence and mental ilness. *Psychiatry* (Edgmont), *5*(5), 34-38.

Sadock, B. J. & Sadock, V. A. (2007). *Kaplan and Sadock's Synopsis of Psychiatry: Behavioral Sciences/Clinical Psychiatry* 10th ed. Philadelphia: Lippincott Williams & Wilkins.

Savolainen, J., Eisman, A., Mason, W. A., Schwartz, J. A., Miettunen, J. & Järvelin, M. R. (2018). Socioeconomic disadvantage and psychological deficits: pathways from early cumulative risk to late-adolescent criminal conviction. *J Adolesc*, 2018, 65, 16–24.

Schreiber, L. R. N., Grant, J. E. & Odlaug, B. L. (2012). Emotion regulation and impulsivity in young adults. *J Psychiatr Res*, *46*, 651–58.

Scott, D. (2008). *Toolkit for Primary Care: Capacity. Regional Geriatric.* London: Program of SW Ontario Parkwood Hospital.

Slater, D. & Hans, V. P. (1984). Public opinion of forensic psychiatry following the Hinckley verdict. *Am J Psychiatry*, *141*, 675-9.

Soysal, H. (2012). Adli Psikiyatri. İstanbul: Özgür Yayınları.

Stams, G. J., Brugman, D., Deković, M., van Rosmalen, L., van der Laan, P. & Gibbs, J. C. (2006). The moral judgment of juvenile delinquents: a meta-analysis. *J Abnorm Child Psychol*, *34*, 692-708.

Steinberg, L. (2004). Risk taking in adolescence: what changes, and why? *Ann N Y Acad Sci*, *1021*, 51-8.

Steinberg, L. (2005). Cognitive and affective development in adolescence. *Trends Cogn Sci*, *9*, 69-74.

Taskıran, S., Mutluer, T., Tufan, A. E. & Semerci, B. (2017). Understanding the associations between psychosocial factors and severity of crime in juvenile delinquency: a cross-sectional study. *Neuropsychiatr Dis Treat*, *18*(13), 1359-66.

Turan Yurtsever, N. (2019). *Forensic Psychiatry. The Studies of Current Health Sciences I.* Ankara: Akademisyen Publisher.

Ural, C., Oncu, F. 7 Belli, H ve Soysal H. (2013). Violent behavior variables among patients with schizophrenia under forensic psychiatric process: a case-control study. *Turk Psikiyatri Derg*, *24*(1), 17-24

Volovka, J. (2013) Violence in schizophrenia and bipolar disorders. *Psychiatr Danub*, *25*, 24-33.

Volavka, J. & Swanson, J. (2010). Violent behavior in mental illness: the role of substance abuse. *JAMA*, *304*, 563-564.

Wallace, C., Mullen, P., Burgess, P., Palmer, S., Ruschena, D. & Browne, C. (1998). Serious criminal offending and mental disorder. *Br J Psychiatry*, *172*, 477-84.

Williams-Evans, S. A. & Myers, J. S. (2004). Adolescent violence. *ABNF J*, *15*(2), 31-34.

Yee, N. Y. L., Large, M. M., Kemp, R. I. & Nielssen, O. B. (2011). Severe non-lethal violence during psychotic illness. *Aust N Z J Psychiatry*, *45*, 466-72.

Yıldız, A. (2018). The effect of neuroanatomic development in childhood and adolescents to the juvenile criminal responsibility. *Adli Tıp Bülteni*, *23* (3), 190-200.

Yoon, J. H., Kim, J. H., Choi, S. S., Lyu, M. K., Kwon, J. H., et al. (2012). Homicide and bipolar I disorder: A 22-year study. *Forensic Science International*, *217*, 113–118.

Yu, R., Geddes, J. R. & Fazel, S. (2012). Personality disorders, violence, and antisocial behavior: a systematic review and meta-regression analysis. *J Personal Disord*, *26*(5), 775-92.

In: Forensic Psychiatry …
Editor: Nursen Turan Yurtsever
ISBN: 978-1-53619-530-9

Chapter 3

OFFENDER PROFILE

Sinem Yıldız İnanıcı*
Department of Medical Education,
Marmara University School of Medicine, Istanbul, Turkey

ABSTRACT

Profiling is making inferences about the possible characteristics of an offender from the available data. Despite its popularity among the public and use by law enforcement in investigations, the legal definition of *profiler*, the skills a profiler should have, and the scientific validity of profiling methods are still debated. The lack of legal definitions can be related to the inability to follow practices to a certain standard and the continuing uncertainty regarding the ethical responsibilities. The fact that the profiling process includes uncertainties due to its nature can make the process vulnerable to errors that may cost individuals their rights and freedoms. A profiler should be under an obligation to be aware of the scientific bases he uses, be able to reflect on the cognitive biases, be aware of the weaknesses of the data and methods he uses, and bear a professional and ethical responsibility. The generalizability of the research results can be strenthened by adding more profilers to the studies investigating the effectiveness of profiling. It is essential to create a scientific description of

* Corresponding Author's E-mail: yildiz.sinem@gmail.com.

the competencies that a profiler should have and directly measure these competencies in research. Institutions that use profiling can prevent rights violations if they establish their ethical guidelines and ensure that they are followed. In this paper, the problems faced by profilers who reason and make decisions to evaluate complex criminal behavior are described in the context of psychological biases and ethical principles.

DEFINITION

Profiling is an attempt to bring together the available evidence through observation and reflection to solve a criminal event and prevent recidivism. The specific purpose of profiling is to reveal the perpetrator's personality traits, discover the unique patterns in the way the criminal commits the crime, and, if possible, reveal the motivation for the crime (Kocsis and Palermo 2007). In the profiling process, data such as evidence obtained from the crime scene and autopsy results are collected and sent to the profiler to estimate possible personality, behavioral, and demographic characteristics. Then the profile is transmitted to the units conducting the investigation (Hicks and Sales 2006).

Profiling serves in various processes within the criminal justice system. During the investigation phase, especially when traditional research methods fail, it aims to associate crimes committed at different times, identify the characteristics of the unknown criminal, identify the behavioral patterns that the criminal may show before and after committing a crime, and determine the predictions and tactics for preventing recidivism. Profiling in the apprehension process aims to predict the criminal's reactions to the arrest and make suggestions to improve the prosecution. The profiler can also act as an expert in court to associate the crime and the criminal during the trial process (Hicks and Sales 2006).

As it is understood, profiling is an inferential process in which many variables related to the crime are taken into account (Petherick 2003). The criminal sketch created by the profiler should be a trained guess based on evidence, victimology, and scientific theory (Geberth 1996). The profiler develops an idea about the unknown person or people by establishing a working hypothesis regarding a particular crime based on the available data and proven theories, which is the opposite of profiling already known people such as artists and politicians (Turco 2008).

The fact that profiling includes many psychological, investigative, and legal variables and aims to reach an unknown person can make this process open to error. Thus, although profiling is a valuable tool in detecting criminals, it has its limitations and is recommended for use with other reliable investigation techniques (Geberth 1996).

THEORETICAL APPROACHES IN OFFENDER PROFILING

Diagnostic Evaluations

After the contribution of a psychiatrist in the cases of the Mad Bomber of New York City and Boston Strangler of Boston (for the cases see Alison 2005), the role of the psychologist and psychiatrist in the clarification of cases began to differ. These people began to be summoned to the courts for investigations for purposes other than assessing the criminal's mental health. Experiences of such cases have led expert researchers to start to pay attention to the use of abnormal psychology and clinical evaluation processes to solve the cases (Geberth 1996).

Kocsis (2010) reports that this old form of profiling is not a defined approach. Experts analyze criminal behavior and make predictions about the criminal based on their training and clinical experience in their field.

Criminal Investigative Analysis

The inadequacy of both diagnostic assessment and classical investigative methods has led to the development of the criminal investigative analysis (CIA). CIA defines profiling as one of the forensic investigative techniques used within a policing context (Kocsis 2010).

Hazelwood and Douglas (1980) implemented the CIA's typological approach based on their experience and literature. The authors define lust murder separately from sadistic homicide as it involves mutilation and displacement of the genitals. The authors divide the perpetrators of this crime into two classes—organized nonsocial and disorganized asocial. According to this classification, the organized person is insensitive to society, irresponsible,and egocentric. He does not avoid people even though he does not like them, is methodological, realizes that his action is a crime and recognizes its effects on society, and lives a certain distance from the crime scene. The disorganized type avoids social relations and has difficulty in interpersonal relationships, feels less methodological, feels isolated, and chooses the crime location closer to her job or home. This process, which started with Hazelwood and Douglas (1980), continues todevelop more detailed and comprehensive manuals that include different crimes (Dougles et al. 2013).

The typological approach has clarified the evidence collection and evaluation processes. On the other hand, there are many variables within a proposed typology, and their interaction and interpretation of these variables require a more systematic approach (Kocsis 2010).

Investigative Psychology

Investigative psychology (IP) covers all aspects of the different fields of psychology related to civil or criminal investigations. It integrates psychological knowledge into the processes of managing, investigating, and convicting the criminal. In this approach, profiling is not only considered as a technique. It is also aimed to develop theoretical, methodological, and practical models that can be used to solve the crime. Testing the inferences to be made about the criminal from the crime scene and basing on evidence is prioritized (Canter 2000).

It is essential to model the inferential processes used to make inferences about the criminal's characteristics from what is known to the police about the criminal. One can use personality theory approaches related to social context and crime scene analyses to model these processes, but each has its strengths and weaknesses (Canter and Gregory 1994).

Multi-dimensional scaling (MDS) is frequently used to analyze crime behaviors and other characteristic offender behavior in this approach (Kocsis 2010). MDS can examine the relationship between many variables and express the correlations between variables in a diagram form. These diagrams are usually square, and the variables are icons in the square. Each icon's location and placement in the square show the relationship between variables. While the icons' proximity indicates a strong relationship between them, a third variable standing away from these two variables in the square diagram is unrelated or weakly related to the first two (Kocsis 2006).

Behavioral Evidence Analysis

In the behavioral evidence analysis (BEA) approach, evaluating the extensive behavioral evidence related to the crime over time reveals the criminal-specific correlations, motives, and predispositions. While some features do not change much throughout the criminal career, some may differ depending on the situation (Turvey 2012).

The BEA uses an ideo-deductive method that evaluates and interprets physical evidence such as shoe traces, blood spatter patterns, fingerprints, injuries, and toxicological testing results (Mateescu and Ipate 2016) and victimology and crime scene characteristics such as method of approach, method of attack, method of control, and location type. As a result of examining these units one by one, an analysis is conducted to reveal behavioral patterns. Analyzing the crime scene or criminal profile in this way is necessarily based on the evidence supporting the result obtained from the analysis (Mateescu and Ipate 2016). The use of critical thinking, scientific method, and analytical logic is essential (Turvey 2012).

Since the perpetrator learns and changes like other people, behavioral evidence analysis is not a method that gives fixed results, but it is an ongoing, dynamic, and analytical process. The profiler should have critical thinking skills that allow him to handle cases objectively and methodologically and be aware of his personality traits and possible interference with the offender's evaluations while revealing his characteristics to be alert to intuition bias (Mateescu and Ipate 2016).

Crime Action Profiling

Crime action profiling (CAP) is very similar to CIA. Still, it uses statistical techniques such as MDS to develop models "in which crime behaviors are correlated with various offender characteristics and thus operate as mechanisms by which the perpetrators of future crimes may be profiled" (Kocsis 2009, p. 220).

Unlike CIA, CAP is described as a technique that works in forensic psychology/psychiatry, not policing. CAP research and practices are based on developing crime profile models and concerned with the effectiveness of criminal profiling processes and the related logistic factors. CAP, like IP, uses MDS but does not do so by running a separate analysis of data on criminal behavior and criminal characteristics. It uses MDS to create models that can guide making predictions using other statistical and mathematical tools (Kocsis 2010).

Despite claims to be successful in some cases, post hoc evaluations of created profiles weaken their power. Regardless of its method, profiling in a legal context continues to struggle to become a scientific practice (Norris and Petherick 2010).

Validity and Reliability of the Methods in Offender Profiling

It is a multidimensional and complex issue to draw a quality picture that will significantly contribute to identifying the criminal by profiling. Topics such as the unclear definition of a profiler, scientific validity of the techniques and assumptions, the validity of the evidence used in profiling, and the nature of human reasoning and decision-making mechanisms can make it more difficult to profile.

The validity of profiling, that is, its accuracy in correctly predicting an unknown offender's characteristics, and its usefulness depend on the scientific evaluation of each issue and increasing the practitioner's awareness on these issues. Observations and studies on profiling so far have implications for the development of scientific perspective on this issue.

Definition of the Profiler

The definition of a criminal profiler as a specialty and the profiler's qualificationsare not clearly defined (Snook et al. 2008). This definition's absence or ambiguity makes it difficult to determine what qualifications profilers should have and what formal training they should receive (Norris and Petherick 2010). Kocsis and Coleman (2000) also report that in most countries, profiling practices are not regulated by legal forces in a way to establish sound practice principles and eliminate unethical elements. There is still a long way to go so that this evolving discipline's contributions can be used safely in court (Norris and Petherick 2010).

Failure to set professional standards in profiling, as in any discipline, causes significant differences in practitioners' skills. The observation of such differences among those investigating criminal incidents can have negative implications for justice achievement (Innes 2003).

A series of studies have been conducted to determine the profiler's qualities and the characteristics that distinguish the profiler from the other specialists. Pinizzotto and Finkel (1990) compared expert profilers' performances with police detectives, clinical psychologists, and undergraduate students. In the study, the participants read a closed murder case and a closed sexual crime case. The researchers examined what the participants remembered about the case, the details they saw important in the case, their predictions about who the perpetrator might be, and their reasons. Profilers prepared richer reports for both cases than other groups. All groups remembered more details about the sex crime case, although the profilers and psychologists provided more details. Other detectives evaluated the usefulness of the profiles written by the participants. Accordingly, the most beneficial profile for investigation was the profile prepared by the experts/teachers who were experienced and taught profiling. Professional profilers' reports came in second place. The ratio of correctly detecting offender characteristics of all groups was higher than chance. In the sex offense case, the analysisshowed that profilers scored significantly better than the other three groups combined. In the line-up process for a sex offense, the expert/teachers were accurate in identifying the offender 100 percent of the time, and the profilers were accurate 83 percent of the time. Accuracy was lower for the other groups. The participants did not show the same detection difference for homicide. Profilers indicated significantly more details as necessary and important than non-profilers for both cases.

Kocsis et al. (2000) compared a profiler group with police, psychologists, students, and psychic groups using a closed homicide case. The participants read the case, made detailed descriptions of the offender, and filled in a thirty-three-item questionnaire. The questionnaire contained the dimensions of offender characteristics, cognitions related to the offense, behaviors related to the offense, and the offender's personal history. Then they used adjectives to describe the psychological aspects of the offender. The groups did not differ significantly in total accuracy scores and in using adjectives to describe the offender's psychological properties. Psychologists performed better than police in physical characteristics and offense behavior dimensions. In the analysis performed by dividing the groups into two as profiler and non-profiler, the profiler group's total accuracy and cognitive process subdimension scores were higher than the non-profiler ones.

In another study, Kocsis (2003) analyzed the content of the profiler reports that profilers wrote about a murder case with groups similar to those in the previous research and found that the profiler reports were longer than the non-profiler ones. Profilers' reports contained more information about the offender's nonphysical descriptive features and the crime or the behavior of the offender before, during, and after the crime. All groups provided an equal number of physical descriptors of the offender.

When Kocsis (2004) compared the profiler's performance with police detective, fire investigator, control group, and science students, he found that the groups differed significantly on the total number of questions correct. Profilers answered more questions correctly than police detectives. There was no difference between the four sub-measures (i.e., physical features, cognitive processes, offense, behaviors, and social history and habits). However, differences in the social history and habits measure were marginally significant. Professional profilers and science students answered more questions correctly than the group given no information about the case. The professional profilers answered more questions correctly on all except the offense behavior subdimension. The science students consistently ranked second to the profilers except for the offense behaviors sub-measure, in which they excelled. However, the profilers' performance was not statistically distinct from the science students across any of the measures. On the other hand, professional profilers were statistically better than the police detectives on the total accuracy measure and social history and habits sub-measure. Among the groups, the fire investigators' and police detectives' performances were not better than the control group who relied on the social stereotype to construct the profile.

Although Kocsis's studies say something about the skills of professional profilers, they are open to criticism. It has been criticized that the questionnaire used in the studies may produce different answers according to the person who answered the items. For example, one of these items was related to the offender's height, and the options were very short, average, etc. It may be misleading to consider qualitatively very different groups (student, psychic, etc.) as a single group in the mentioned studies and report that the profiler's performances are better than these because the non-offender group is not homogeneous in itself. Because the profilers make a better profile than another group does not prove that their profile is more accurate in reality. The researchers should look at the profilers' performances against the absolute criteria that define useful profiling. Also, the length of the profile reports does not prove that they are also high in accuracy. To determine what skills are necessary and vital in profiling, operational descriptions of these skills should be made, and skills should be measured directly. However, Kocsis used science students to represent analytical and critical thinking skills in his studies, while psychics represent intuition. Also, more than one skill can coexist in a group or a person. Bennell et al. (2006) measured critical thinking skills with a scale in which participants completed a mock profiling exercise. They found no relationship between profile accuracy scores and critical thinking scores.

Also, the number of profilers participating in the studies is minimal. Getting evaluations by isolating the participants and using multiple-choice questionnaires is not suitable for real-life profiling conditions. Profiling is typically an interactive process and involves exchanging people's ideas from different disciplines (Bennell et al. 2006).

The Reliability of the Data Used in Profiling

The reliability of the data used by a profiler in the evaluation process also plays an essential role in inferring the potential offender characteristics. Incorrect collection of these data or lack of evidence can mislead the process.

The information provided by those who witnessed a crime is used as evidence to solve the case and draw conclusions about the offender's characteristics. However, the reliability of the information given by the witness is also affected by many factors. Wells, Memon, and Penrod (2006) summarize these factors as follows: People may be more prone to making mistakes in identifying people who belong to a different race than themselves. Also, the level of stress that can be caused by witnessing the event can negatively affect the identification accuracy and eyewitness recall. High stress can disrupt both processes. The stress experienced during questioning can negatively affect recognition and recall. Besides, weapon focus, directing the witness's attention sources to the attack weapon, may cause her not to process other details about the event sufficiently and, therefore, to remember or misrecognize. How long the witness was exposed to the incident, whether the attacker was disguised, and length of time between the date of the crime and testifying will also affect the eyewitness information quality. Whether or not the eyewitness is under the influence of alcohol or asubstance during the incident is another disruptive factor to consider.

Both the law enforcement who provide information to the profiler and the profiler can naturally use stereotypes when approaching evidence. Stereotypes are generalizations about those belonging to a group or social category. They speed up and simplify judgment and perception but are often exaggerated, negative, and not open to change, even if there is evidence against them (Americal Psychological Association 2020, November 8).

Although stereotypes are part of the human mind's natural function, those involved in the profiling process should prevent them from becoming prejudices. It is essential that profiling is based on apparent evidence-based behaviors, but stereotypes are related to how behavior is perceived internally. For example, the intrusion of prejudice on issues such as a suspect's race (Lee et al. 2007), socioeconomic status, and occupation in a labeling manner may wear down the evaluation process.

The law enforcement and the profilers may be under stress due to their professions'demands and the crime at hand. If they cannot manage this stress, negative consequences may be reflected in the crime evaluation process. Even in routine civilian crime scene investigations, practitioners' stress levels increase (Adderley et al. 2012). The illumination of child murders is perceived as more complex and demanding than adult murders and may cause more emotional stress than adult murders (Roach Cartwrightand Sharatt 2017). Other factors that increase stress and make the process open to error include fear of the possibility that law enforcement will make mistakes and lose the case and that their mistakes are more open to the public than other justice professionals (Clark et al. 2015).

The Reliability of the Underlying Theory and Assumptions

Generally, the underlying assumption of profiling is that one can predict future crimes by looking at past crimes. However, Kocsis and Palermo

(2007) warn that there is a problem in sample representation in the studies and the accuracy of the data used. For example, the typologies in the work of Ressler et al. (1986) have been criticized for involving interviews with a small number of and only detained criminals. In another study challenging the typology approach, Canter et al. (2004) examined the co-occurrence patterns of thirty-nine traits in murders committed by a hundred serial killers. MDS did not indicate any specific subsets of offender characteristics related to organized-disorganized typologies in this study. In contrast, organized features have been more common in most serial murders than disorganized ones.

The typology-based approaches used in profiling contain several basic assumptions: The first of these assumptions is the so-called homology assumption. Accordingly, criminals with similar criminal behavior show similar characteristics. Another premise involves the idea that the criminal shows consistency for each of his crimes. The third assumption, behavioral differentiation, is that a criminal's behavior must be distinctly different from the behavior of another criminal (Canter 2000; Mokros and Alison 2002).

However, the homology assumption is not supported by scientific studies. Bateman and Salfati (2007) described thirty-five offender behaviors in 450 cases committed by ninety criminals. The authors examined the frequency of each of these behaviors and the themes they formed from these behaviors (planning and control behavior, mutilation behavior, sexual behavior, stealing behavior, and gun behavior) in the events committed by each criminal and how consistently they were displayed. Thus, they were able to evaluate the effectiveness of both individual behaviors and category usage. The results showed that neither of the approaches were useful in distinguishing serial murders committed by a single criminal and a criminal may not behave consistently in different cases. Doan and Snook (2008) tested whether a classification made using arson and robbery data in a region can be used for crimes in another geographic area. The results indicated that ready-made typologies could not be easily used to classify the crimes at hand. The homology assumption was not confirmed in more than half of the cases. Mokros and Alison (2002) evaluated age, sociodemographic characteristics, and a previous criminal conviction in their study with a hundred British stranger rapist samples, but the homology assumption was not supported. Bennell et al. (2013) examined the usefulness of another typology by examining fifty-three serial sexual murder cases with proximity scaling. Still, they could not find any evidence for the co-occurrence of offender behaviors they identified.

Turvey (2012) also states that profiling assumptions do not reflect criminal behavior's multifaceted nature and that criminals can show the same behavior with very different motivations. Personality theory approaches even challenge the belief that a person will behave consistently in separate crimes. Although individuals can demonstrate a degree of consistency in their behavior, the degree of this consistency depends on the psychological similarity of the situations in which the behavior occurs. In addition to this psychological similarity, other factors must be considered when evaluating the assumption of consistency. One of these factors may be that the behavior is automated or absorbed by the person. Consistency in this type of behavior is more likely than a planned action. The person demonstrates behavior that he or she specializes inmore consistently, and the behaviors shown in short time intervals show higher consistency with each other (Woodhams Hollin and Bull 2007).

It is crucial to understand the physical similarity of some aspects in the case and what these elements mean for the criminal when using profiling. Different features may be the result of the same perception of offenders. It may be necessary to understand what offense behaviors the offender might have mastered and remember that there may be changes in offender perception and behavior in the period between these events if there is more than one event. Different elements may be the result of the same perception of offenders.

Studies on the validity and usefulness of profiling are also criticized. Chifflet (2015) suggests that determining how close the profiler's predictions are to the sentenced perpetrator's characteristics can be used to test the validity. Accordingly, in a large sample, the criminal's attributes can be listed in detail, and by looking at which ones are detected in the profile, the accuracy of the profile can be reached. However, Alison et al. (2003), in their study of twenty-one profiles, found that almost a quarter of the claims in the reports were ambiguous and about half were unprovable. Less than a third were prone to falsifiability.

Fergusson (2009) says that for a profile to be investigatively relevant, it must contain the following attributes: (1) It should not include expressions that are used to distinguish the offender from the general population or the criminal population, such as saying that the offender is married in a profile. (2) It should eliminate the expressions that would not help progress in the conduct of the investigation, such as the offender's mother being dominant or having sexual problems. (3) It should not mention the offender features unless there is substantial and reliable evidence, and it should allow them to speak on their behalf if there are characteristics supported by the evidence. (4) The evaluation should include the offender's behavior and the inferences made about the offender from these behaviors. Also, it is essential to link these inferences with the evidence at the crime scene.

Tversky and Kahneman (1974) report that individuals rely on limited heuristics when performing complex tasks such as evaluating and predicting probability. While these heuristics are beneficial, they can also cause serious errors (Risinger and Loop 2002). It should be kept in mind that people are open to an error by using these shortcuts in evaluating and probabilistic processes, such as profiling, where there is uncertainty in many aspects.

Perceived Contribution of Offender Profiling

Views on the usefulness of profiling in the field are discussed to assess profiling's validity and utility. However, law enforcement opinions about the validity and effectiveness of profiling are also influenced by many factors. Kocsis and Hayes (2004) gave a profile to police officers and reported to one group that an expert profiler made the profile. Another group was informed that an unspecified author prepared it. They found that when it was said that expert profilers made the profile, there was a perception that the offender was determined with higher accuracy. On the other hand, the perceptions about the usefulness of the profile in solving the case were not affected by the profiler's quality.

Trager and Brewster (2001) sent their questionnaires about the psychological profile's effectiveness to ninety-six police departments in the USA; forty-six departments responded. Thirty-seven percent of these departments reported that they do not use psychological profiling. The psychological profile is mostly used in rape and murder cases, and the profilers are often FBI profilers and lead detectives. Researchers questioned the usefulness of psychological profiling for interrogation strategies, directing the investigation, predicting future behavior, and identifying a suspect. The rate of reporting that psychological profiling helps the investigation process varied between 37.8 percent and 62.2 percent. The participants' ratio of thinking that psychological profiling is neither harmful nor beneficial varied between 28.9 percent and 40.5 percent. The rate of thinking that psychological profiling is useful is highest for developing inquiry strategies. It is mostly rated as neither helpful nor unhelpful in determining the offender's future behavior.

Snook et al. (2007) interviewed fifty-one police officers about their experiences with criminal profiling and beliefs about its usage. Officers mostly agreed that criminal profiling contributes to the cases' solutions and improves the investigators' understanding of the cases. A certain number of officers suggested that information that the profiler providescan be usedas evidence. In addition, they saw no risk of being misdirected by the profiler and felt that utilizing a profiling technique is appropriate regardless of the offense type.

Torres, Boccaccini, and Miller (2006) conducted an internet survey of 161 forensic psychologists and psychiatrists. Approximately one-third of the participants stated that they know about profiling, 16.3 percent of the participants received training on profiling, and 10.9 percent have generated a profile for an investigation. Approximately one-fifth of the participants found it scientifically valid in associating the suspect with a crime, 17.1 percent found it scientifically reliable, and about one-third found it scientifically supported enough to be used in court under any circumstances.

A meta-analysis indicates no scientific evidence to support the public's positive view of criminal profiling. Many criminal profiling approaches do not use evidence-based typologies and old theories of human behavior (Snook et al.2007).

Ethical Considerations

The uncertainties mentioned above and controversial issues regarding profiling make this area open to some unethical practices. Turvey (2012) states that because the profiler is not professionally defined, people who describe themselves as a profiler cannot be officially held responsible. They can be comfortable acting irresponsibly. Whatever specialization a profiler has, he needs to conceptualize his role in the investigation. If a profiler feels responsible only for his academic or scientific goals, he may ignore the requirement that his opinions in profiling must have validity.

Ethical guidelines of professions involved in profiling can help determine the general principles of profiling practices. A profiler must first act in a way that guarantees the rights and welfare of those he contacts professionally and other related people and must be aware of his responsibility to society. He should improve accuracy, truthfulness, and honesty in his practice and express the proven facts in a simple way (APA 2010). He must not misrepresent case data and scientific principles that he used to interpret the evidence. To preserve the principles of honesty and objectivity (American Academy of Psychiatry and the Law 2005), the profiler should be aware of the possible biases and limitations of the field of expertise when reaching the offender characteristics (APA 2010; AAPL 2005).

More specifically, a professionalshould clear the ethical conflict that may arise between legal authorities and present his competence within his education, training, and the supervision he received (APA 2010; AAPL 2005). Moreover, he should take reasonable steps to ensure his work's competence in profiling, where adequate training requirements are ambiguous. If there is personal, scientific, legal, or financial conflict of interest that impairsa professional's objectivity and exposes the people or organizations to harm, he should refrain from taking a professional role in the case (APA 2010). He is also responsible for taking precautions regarding confidentiality and should not disclose personally identifiable information (APA 2010; AAPL 2005).

Based on the principles mentioned above, Turvey (2012) suggests that profilers should adhere to the role of an instructor providing objective and scientific knowledge without alarming the public or creating sensations while consulting media-related projects. Before making a statement about a case, a profiler should decide whether he is qualified to explain a particular case, whether there is enough publicly available information to give an idea, and whether the ideas he shares will harm the investigation process. Suppose a profiler sees the media attention as a professional validation tool and wants to keep that interest alive. In that case, his statements to the media run the risk of not complying with ethical principles. A profiler should act by taking into account the people's rights and freedoms in his publications in both memoirs and other forms (Turvey 2012).

Kocsis and Coleman (2000) warn practitioners of various misuses of the criminal psychological profile. One of these misuses is assuming a person is guilty only because he fits the profile. Just as the presence of someone's fingerprints on the scene does not make him guilty, the person's fit to a profile cannot be definitive proof of guilt. A profile only presents a probability. The fact that someone does not fit a profile does not mean that the person is innocent. The fact that the profile does not give precise information about the person's characteristics prevents innocence attribution. It is a misuse for the reasons mentioned above that a suspect's characteristics are presented as evidence in court and evaluated as definitive evidence of guilt. There may be situations where a suspect fits well into a profile, but there is no evidence that the person is guilty. In such a situation, especially a profiler who does not have sufficient law experience, being too involved in the case may make himmisconstruethe profile. Putting too much emphasis on psychological profiling can prevent a suspect from being arrested if the profile is wrong, or the suspect may not be adequately investigated by the police simply because a suspect does not fit the profile. Organizations that use offender profiling should establish specific ethical codes to protect ethical values, priorities, and implementation standards and control their implementation (Turvey 2012).

CONCLUSION

Defining the profiler and determining the skills that a profiler should have based on evidence are necessary for standardizing the practices and ensuring ethical practices. In a profiler's education, reflective training and reflective practice should be provided to minimize the risk of people falling into cognitive biases. Institutions can be encouraged to present their explanations on the effectiveness of this approach based on scientific evidence to regulate profiling's public visibility. Establishing ethical standards that will cover all the elements mentioned above for profilers' practice and ensuring their implementation will contribute to the criminal justice system's effective functioning.

REFERENCES

Adderley, R., Smith, L. L., Bond, J. W., and Smith, M. (2012). Physiological Measurement of Crime Scene Investigator Stress. *International Journal of Police Science & Management*, 14, 166–176.

Alison, L. (Ed.) (2005). *The forensic psychologist's casebook psychological profiling and criminal investigation*. London: Willan Publishing.

Alison, L., Smith, M. D., Eastman, O., and Rainbow, L. (2003). Toulmin's philosophy of argument and its relevance to offender profiling. *Psychology, Crime & Law,* 9, 173–183.

American Academy of Forensic Sciences Bylaws. (n.d.). *Chapter II: Code of ethics.* Retrieved from http://ethics.iit.edu/codes/AAFS%201978.pdf.

American Academy of Psychiatry & the Law. (2020, November 9). *Ethical guidelines for the practice of forensic psychiatry*. Retrieved from https://www.aapl.org/ethics.htm.

American Psychological Association (2020, November 10). *Ethical principles of psychologists and code of conduct.* Retrived from https://www.apa.org/ethics/code/principles.pdf.

Bateman, A. L., and Salfati, C. G. (2007). An examination of behavioral consistency using individual behaviors or groups of behaviors in serial homicide. *Behavioral Sciences & The Law,* 25, 527–544.

Bennell, C., Bloomfield, S., Emeno, K., and Musolino, E. (2013). Classifying serial sexual murder/murderers: An attempt to validate Keppel and Walter's (1999) model. *Criminal Justice and Behavior,* 40, 5–25.

Bennell, C., Jones, N. J., Taylor, P. J., & Snook, B. (2006). Validities and abilities in criminal profiling: a critique of the studies conducted by Richard Kocsis and his colleagues. *International Journal of Offender Therapy and Comparative Criminology,* 50, 344–360.

Canter, D. (2000). Offender profiling and criminal differentiation. *Legal and Criminological Psychology,* 1, 23–46.

Canter, D. (2004). Offender profiling and investigative psychology. *Journal of Investigative Psychology and Offender Profiling, 1*, 1–15.

Canter, D. V., Alison, L. J., Alison, E., and Wentink, N. (2004). The organized/disorganized typology of serial murder: myth or model? *Psychology, Public Policy, and Law,* 10, 293–320.

Canter, D., and Gregory, A. (1994). Identifying the residential location of rapists. *Journal Forensic Science Society,* 34, 169-175.

Chifflet, P. (2015). Questioning the validity of criminal profiling: An evidence-based approach. *Australian and New Zealand Journal of Criminology,* 48, 238–255.

Clark, R. D., Distelrath, C., Vaquera, G. S, Winterich, D., and DeZolt, E. (2015). Critical-incident trauma and crime scene investigation: A review of police organizational challenges and interventions. *Sociology.* 32.

Doan, B., Snook, B.(2008). A failure to find empirical support for the homology assumption in criminal profiling. *Journal of Police and Criminal Psychology,* 23, 61–70.

Douglas, J. E., Burgess, A. W., Burgess, A. G., Ressler, R. K. (2013). *Crime classification manual: A standard system for ınvestigating and classifying violent crime* (3rd ed.). San Francisco, CA: John Wiley & Sons.

Fergusson, C. (2009). Investigative relevance. In P. Wayne (Ed.). *Serial Crime Theoretical and Practical Issues in Behavioral Profiling* (2nd ed.). London: Elsevier Academic Press.

Geberth, V. J. (1996). *Practical homicide investigation: Tactics, procedures, and forensic techniques* (4th ed.). Boca Raton, FL: CRC Press.

Hazelwood, R. R. and Douglas, J. E. (1980). The lust murderer. *FBI Law Enforcement Bulletin,* 49, 18-22.

Hicks, S. J. and Sales, B. D. (2006). *Criminal profiling: Developing an effective science and practice.* Washington, DC: American Psychological Association.

Innes, B. (2003). *Profile of a Criminal Mind.* Leicester, UK: Silverdale Books.

Kocsis, R. N. (2003). An emprical assessment of content in criminal psychological profiles. *International Journal of Offender Therapy and Comparative Criminology,* 47, 37-46.

Kocsis, R. N. (2004). Psychological profiling of serial arson offenses. An assessment of skills and accuracy. *Criminal Justice and Behavior,* 31, 341-361.

Kocsis, R. N. (2006). *Criminal profiling principles and practice*. Totowa, New Jersey: Humana Press,

Kocsis, R. N. (2010). Schools of thought related to criminal profiling. In R. N, Kocsis, (Ed.) *Criminal profiling international theory, research, and practice* (2nd ed.) (pp. 393-404). New Jersey: Humana Press.

Kocsis, R. N. (ed.) (2009). *Applied criminal psychology: A guide to forensic behavioral sciences.* Springfield: Charles C. Thomas.

Kocsis, R. N., and Palermo, G. B. (2007). Contemporary problems in criminal profiling. In R. N. Kocsis (Ed.), *Criminal profiling: International theory, research, and practice* (pp. 327–345). New Jersey: Humana Press.

Kocsis, R. N., Irwin, H. J., Hayes, A. F., and Nunn, R. (2000). Expertise in psychological profiling: A comparative assessment. *Journal of Interpersonal Violence, 15*(3), 311-331.

Kocsis, R. N. and Coleman, S. (2000). The unexplored ethics of criminal psychological profiling. In M. G. Godwin (Ed.) *Criminal psychology and forensic technology: A collaborative approach to effective profiling* (pp. 323–338). New York: CRC Press.

Lee, Y. T., Bumgarner, J., Widner, R., and Luo, Z. L. (2007). Psychological models of stereotyping and profiling in law enforcement: How to increase accuracy by using more non-racial cues, *Journal of Crime and Justice,* 30, 87-129.

Mateescu, O. and Ipate, I. (2016). Applying psychological profiling in the investigation of violent offenses. *Behavioral evidence analysis. The international conference education and creativity for a knowledge-based society* (pp.90-95). Vienna, Osterreichish Rumanischer Akademischer Verein.

Mokros, A. and Alison, L. J. (2002). Is offender profiling possible? testing the predicted homology of crime scene actions and background characteristics in a sample of rapists. *Legal and Criminological Psychology*, 7,25-43.

Norris, G. and Petherick, W. (2010). Criminal profiling in the courtrooms: Behavioral investigative advice or bad character evidence. *Cambrian Law Review,* 41, 39-54.

Petherick, W. A. (2003). What's in a name? Comparing applied profiling methodologies. *Journal of Law and Social Challenges,* 5, 173-188.

Pinizzotto, A. J. and Finkel, N. J. (1990). Criminal personality profiling: An outcome and process study. *Law and Human Behavior,* 14, 215-233.

Ressler, R. K., Burgess, A. W., Souglas, J. E., Hartman, C. R. and D'Agostino, R. B. (1986). Sexual killers and their victims: Identifying patterns through crime scene analysis. *Journal of Interpersonal Violence*, 1, 288-308.

Risinger, D. M. and Loop, J. L. (2002). Three card monte, monthly hall, modus operandi and “offender profiling”: some lessons of modern cognitive science for the law of evidence. *Cardozo Law Review,* 24, 193-285.

Roach, J., Cartwright, A. J. J. and Sharatt, K. (2017) The effects of investigating homicide on police investigators. *Journal of Investigating Child Death*, 3, 38-50.

Snook, B., Cullen, R. M., Bennell, C., Taylor, P. J., and Gendreau, P. (2008). The criminal profiling illusion: What’s behind the smoke and mirrors? *Criminal Justice and Behavior,* 35, 1257–1276.

Snook, B., Eastwood, J., Gendreau, P., Goggin, C., and Cullen, R. M. (2007). Taking stock of criminal profiling: A narrative review and meta-analysis. *Criminal Justice and Behavior, 34*(4), 437–453.

Snook, B., Haines, A., Taylor, P. J., and Bennell, C. (2007). Criminal profiling belief and use: A study of Canadian police officer opinion. *Canadian Journal of Police and Security Services, 5.*

Torres, A. N., Boccaccini, M. T., and Miller, H. A. (2006). Perceptions of the validity and utility of criminal profiling among forensic psychologists and psychiatrists. *Professional Psychology: Research and Practice,* 37, 51–58.

Trager, J. and Brewster, J. (2001). The effectiveness of psychological profiles. *Journal of Police Criminal Psychology,* 16, 20–28.

Turco, R. (2008). Criminal Profile Construction and Investigative Procedures Study of the Westley Dodd Serial Sexual Murders. In R. N, Kocsis, (ed.) *Serial murder and the psychology of violent crimes* (2nd ed.) (pp.245-258). New Jersey: Humana Press.

Turvey, B. E. (2012). *Criminal profiling: An introduction to behavioral evidence analysis. London.* UK: Elsevier.

Tversky, A. and Kahneman, D. (1974). Judgment under uncertainty: Heuristics and biases. *Science*, 185, 1124-1131.

Wells, G. L., Memon, A., and Penrod, S. D. (2006). Eyewitness Evidence: Improving its Probative Value. *Psychological Science in the Public Interest,* 7, 45–75.

Woodhams, J., Hollin, C. R., and Bull, R. (2007). The psychology of linking crimes: A review of the evidence. *Legal and Criminological Psychology,* 12, 233–249.

In: Forensic Psychiatry …
Editor: Nursen Turan Yurtsever

ISBN: 978-1-53619-530-9

Chapter 4

VICTIM PROFILE

Süleyman Serhat Gürpinar* and Abdulkadir Yildiz
Department of Forensic Medicine, Faculty of Medicine,
Suleyman Demirel University, Isparta, Turkey

ABSTRACT

Studies conducted on the contributing factors of violence have focused on the personality and the mental, cultural, socioeconomic, and educational characteristics of the perpetrators. In the hopes of preventing violence, precedence has been given to solving problems in the characteristics of these perpetrators. Studies have also been carried out on certain characteristics of victims, but these studies have not been highlighted excessively because it has been inferred that the victim might be an accomplice or even a provocateur in some violent situations. It is possible that perpetrators might use this idea as a line of defense in the case against violence. In addition, in many cultures, there is the belief that the inflicted violence is deserved or that some problems can only be solved by violence. If the contribution of victims in violent cases is brought up, it may help to confirm that these are misguided beliefs. It is also possible to deflect thoughts of victim involvement through today's effective use of social media and the fact that events like this are rarely seen scientifically or

* Corresponding Author's E-mail: serhat.gurpinar@gmail.com.

objectively. However, using a scientific and objective approach, it should be revealed that victims might have characteristics that make them more prone to violence. To prevent violence, it is necessary to deal with both the victim's and perpetrator's profile and to be aware of the importance of eliminating negative factors. With this awareness, providing treatment and rehabilitation to victims to help them escape this profile may contribute to the prevention of violence. With appropriate treatment and support, victims may be able to avoid a perpetrator's violent actions.

INTRODUCTION

Studies related to contributing factors of violence have concentrated on the personality and the mental, cultural, socioeconomic, and educational characteristics of perpetrators. To help prohibit violence, priority has been given to help change these characteristics of the perpetrators. Studies have also investigated the characteristics of the victims, which is another aspect of this issue, yet, studies are rarely brought forward because there is often talk about the victim as an accomplice in or even a provocateur of the violence. Perpetrators can use this assertion in court, and it may be meaningful in their defence in the case of violence. In addition to this, many cultures have beliefs that violence is deserved in some situations or that problems can only be solved by using violence. Stating that the victims have contributed to the violent incidents often leads to these erroneous beliefs. It is also possible to deflect these ideas through the effective use of social media, as the events are rarely looked at scientifically or objectively. Studies concerning the profile of victims have not come far enough to ease these concerns. However, with the increase in violence in all cultures all over the world, we understand that the methods of treating, rehabilitating, or punishing these characteristics in perpetrators do not work well. Although we live in an era in which human rights, tolerance, and solidarity discourses are recorded in national and supranational legal documents, violence has not decreased. Just as the violence in interpersonal relationships has not decreased, neither has the violence between communities.

We need to look at the characteristics of victims who endure violence with a scientific and objective approach. In the prevention of violence, it is important to deal with the factors that make up the profile of the victim as well as the perpetrator and recognize the importance of eliminating these characteristics. Providing treatment and rehabilitation to victims with the awareness of removing them from the victim profile may contribute to the prevention of violence. With appropriate treatment and support, victims may eliminate their chances of being attacked. Victims of violence often experience repetitive violence, particularly certain types of violence, and they are more exposed to violence in certain periods of their lives.

People exposed to repetitive violence generally feel guilt due to the genetic burdens from previous generations, the psycho-physiological irregularities experienced by their mothers during pregnancy, and the problems they experienced in their own childhood, adolescence, and adulthood. They might also defend the treatment planning and methods because these feelings of guilt are formed by unconscious processes that they are unaware of. If physicians, allied health personnel, social support workers, lawyers, prosecutors, and judges working with victims in the field are not aware of victim profiles, they may show negligence in directing the victim to the necessary treatment and rehabilitation processes.

When employees working in the field understand the psychological and physiological mechanisms by which the victims become the target of perpetrators, they will be able to direct them to treatment and contribute to the avoidance of the recurrence of their victimization.

Epigenetic Interaction

Epigenetics refers to the changes in gene expression that involve mitosis and/or meiosis in the chromatin structure without changes in the primary DNA sequence. It is inherited but is a reversible and dynamic process and is an interface between the genome and lifestyle/environmental impact. DNA methylation, which is the addition of the chemical methyl to DNA, causes the suppression of genes and changes in the expression of the related gene and then histone acetylation causes genes to be activated back (Vaissière, Sawan, and Herceg 2008). Factors such as smoking, alcohol habits, physical activity, obesity, psychological or physical stress, trauma, infectious diseases, environmental pollution, and biorhythm disorders can change our epigenomes. In studies conducted on sire mice who were exposed to alcohol, the offspring were observed to suffer from effects such as a physically weak birth, a high death rate, weakness in the immune system, behavioral anomalies, aggressiveness, risk-taking, and anxiety disorders. It has also been found that children of obese fathers can be born with a larger appetite and a weak sense of satisfaction. These same children can have diabetic problems, even if they are not obese. Genealogical research in this area has revealed that the nutritional environment of not only fathers but also grandfathers plays a role in the health of the offspring. There are also many studies showing that using drugs or stimulants affects the epigenome faster and that it is transferred to children. Children of fathers who have used cocaine have less massive brains than other children; as a result, it causes many learning disabilities. In a study conducted with mice who were exposed to higher levels of physical stress, it was observed that the offspring were more aggressive. In a study of an epigenetic inheritance of fear, father mice were taught to feel scared from a certain smell by giving them a shock with electricity. The offspring of these mice responded to the same smell with fear even though they had not experienced any similar pain after birth. The intergenerational epigenetic basis of neuropsychiatric diseases can be seen in these examples. In fact, it is also believed that epigenetic effects can be beneficial in protecting future generations from environmental risks. The problem is that when there is no real danger, future generations will be hypersensitive, and they will likely suffer from symptoms like anxiety or stress disorders (Burggren 2016; Carone et al. 2010; Dias and Ressler 2014; Finegersh and Homanics 2014; Lambrot et al. 2013; Pembrey et al. 2006).

The symptoms of psychological stress that were experienced by fathers and are seen in their children have also been seen in the children of Holocaust war veterans who have been observed to have higher rates of post-traumatic stress disorder (PTSD), depression, and high blood pressure than other adults. It has been seen that hormones were affected in stressed parents during the war, and their children encountered depression and anxiety in adulthood even though they never experienced similar stressful conditions

(Rouse 2015). It is understood that severe stress triggers the factors that cause continuous changes on gene expression, which then contributes to depression and a change in the chromatin structure at certain genomic locations in the limbic regions of the brain (Nestler 2014). PTSD was found in approximately 30 percent of the children of parents who worked in Iraq and Afghanistan and developed PTSD (Sack 2014). It has been observed that if the parents suffered from PTSD, the probability of the child experiencing PTSD is three times higher than normal. Moreover, this situation occurs even though the child does not know the trauma history that was experienced by the family (Glausiusz 2014). More depression and anxiety were observed in children of parents who experienced trauma during the Cambodian genocide, and suicide rates were higher in children of Australians who were veterans of the Vietnam War compared to the general population (Hughes 2014). Suicide rates among Native American teenagers were found to be ten to nineteen times higher than other American teenagers (Bender 2015). It was also determined that stressed mother rats gave birth prematurely, and their daughters also gave birth prematurely even though they were not under stress. In addition, the grandchildren had shorter pregnancies than their own mothers (Yao et al. 2014). Cortisol, a stress hormone, is secreted in order to reduce the stressor effects of trauma and causes high cortisol levels in the blood. Furthermore, cortisol levels decrease in order to maintain a balance in the body with chronic processes in various neuropsychiatric disorders, especially PTSD and chronic pain and fatigue syndromes. These effects include epigenetic mechanisms. Cortisol levels are low in both those who have experienced trauma and their children (Yehuda and Seckl 2011).

The psychological effects from the burden of epigenetic transfers create an unconscious guilty conscience. It can be extremely difficult for people to be aware of their feelings of guilt, as it depends on the events of previous generations. Feelings of guilt contribute to auto-destructive behavior and create a defenseless physiological structure for the aggression of others.

Prenatal/Pregnancy Period of Mother

In a study, 125 pregnant women whose cortisol was high in their amniotic fluid had babies with high cortisol, and when they were seventeen months old, they showed a cognitive deficiency regardless of their prenatal, obstetric, and socioeconomic factors (Bergman et al. 2010). Babies of mothers who are under extreme and constant stress are premature, underweight, and hyperactive (Weintraub and Verny 2014).

The stress experienced by a mother during pregnancy, like the burdens brought on by epigenetic transmission, also created somatic and psychic burdens on the child. Accordingly, both self-mutilative behaviors and behaviors open to the violence of others were observed in the child.

Childhood and Adolescence

Revictimization

Many studies have revealed a strong relationship between childhood maltreatment and adolescent and/or adult victimization. These experiences lead to a phenomenon called "revictimization" and increase the risk of victimization in the later stages of development (e.g., adolescence and adulthood) (Charak et al. 2018; Charak et al. 2020; Messman-Moore and Long 2003). Some research has shown that multiple experiences of childhood maltreatment increase the risk of revictimization in adulthood (Charak, Eshelman, and Messman-Moore 2019; Charak et al. 2020; Classen, Palesh, and Aggarwal 2005; Widom, Czaja, and Dutton 2008).

Research that was conducted on a large sample of university students showed that women who reported two or more forms of childhood maltreatment were three times more likely to suffer from sexual revictimization than women who reported either one experience of childhood maltreatment or none at all (Jankowski et al. 2002).

In a study on 409 women receiving in-patient treatment that examined the relationship between childhood abuse history and subsequent sexual assault, 45 percent of the participants stated that they were subjected to some form of childhood abuse and 22 percent experienced sexual assault at least once in adulthood. The hierarchical logistic regression analysis, which was appliedafter controlling for sociodemographic and diagnostic variables, showed thatwomen with a history of abuse in childhood are 3.1 times more likely to be sexually assaulted in adulthood than those who have not experienced abuse. Women who have reported physical abuse or both physical and sexual abuse have a higher prevalence of sexual assault in adulthood than women who have reported only sexual abuse. This information shows that physical abuse in childhood is a potential risk factor for sexual assault victimization in adulthood (Cloitre et al. 1996). Nineteen empirical studies, which were defined by at least one sexual abuse victimization in childhood and revictimization of sexual assault in adulthood anddetermined the rate of revictimization and compared it to a sample without revictimization, were analysed in a meta-analytical review. According to these studies, the overall impact size ofrevictimization was confirmed as 59 percent, and it was specified asa moderate effect, which shows a definite relationship between childhood victimization and adult victimization experiences (Roodman and Clum 2001).

In a sample group involving 248 African American and White American women aged eighteen to thirty-six in a study examining sexual revictimization, approximately half of the women who were sexually abused before the age of eighteen faced revictimization of sexual assault in adulthood. Findings of the study showed the presence of a significant relationship between unwanted pregnancy and sexual revictimization and multiple sexual partners and short-term sexual intercourse. These women reported more than one victimization in both their childhood and adulthood (Wyatt, Guthrie, and Notgrass 1992).

In a study involving 1,887 navy women to examine the effects of childhood abuse on subsequent adult abuse, it was found that 57 percent of the participants were exposed to physical and/or sexual abuse in childhood, and women sexually abused in childhood were 4.8 times more likely to be exposed to sexual assault in adulthood when compared to those physically abused in childhood (Merrill et al. 1999).

A study carried out on 341 undergraduate students identified that childhood sexual abuse history directly contributes to sexual victimization in adulthood but that childhood physical abuse also contributes to this risk of victimization (Arata and Lindman 2002).

In addition, in a study of 475 female university students, the highest rate of sexual and/or physical victimization in adulthood was shown by those who suffered both physical and sexual abuse during childhood. The next highest rate was for those who were abused physically in childhood and then those who were sexually abused. The lowest rate applied to those who had never been abused. Significantly high rates of PTSD and trauma symptoms were found in those sexually and physically abused in childhood (Schaaf and McCanne 1998).

There are studies showing that the other forms of maltreatment (negative home environment, neglect, punishment) also increase the risk of victimization in adulthood. Furthermore, diversity of maltreatments increases the probability of victimization in adulthood (Clemmons et al. 2003; Irwin 1999; Sanders and Moore 1999).

In a study of 520 young women born in New Zealand who were followed from their birth to age eighteen, the rate of early onset consensual sexual activity after the age of sixteen, pregnancy at a young age, multiple sexual partners, unprotected sexual intercourse, sexually transmitted diseases, and recurrent sexual victimization were reported statistically significantly higher in young women who reported childhood sexual abuse than those who did not report any abuse (Fergusson, Horwood, and Lynskey 1997).

In a study of 568 university women who reported sexual abuse by incest, someone in their peer group, or adult family members in childhood and those who had never experienced childhood sexual abuse, it was determined that the probability of revictimization of women who were the victims of childhood incest was higher than for those who were abused by a peer or an adult family member. It was also found that revictimization of those who were subjected to childhood sexual abuse by a peer was higher than for those who were sexually abused by nonfamily members. In the same study, depending on the type of sexual abuse in childhood, the shame experienced by the victims was determined to be a statistically significant predictor for revictimization (Kessler and Bieschke 1999).

Psychosocial Development

In a study comparing children who experienced childhood maltreatment with those who did not, it was shown that the history of abuse was the predictor of affect dysregulation, affective lability/negativity, and socially inappropriate emotion expressions in the children. Maltreatment was explained as a mechanism of action above reactive aggression by this emotion dysregulation with poor attention modulation. These situations are major obstacles to the communication between individuals (A. Shields and Cicchetti 1998).

Studies show that physical and/or sexual abuse causes negative behaviour and anger in children aged zero to four, lack of self-control in children aged five to seven, and incompatibility with peers and bullying or bullying victimization in children older than eight years (Erickson, Egeland, and Pianta 1989; Hennessy et al. 1994; Howes and Eldredge 1985; A. M. Shields, Cicchetti, and Ryan 1994). In an analysis of forty-five studies, it was determined that sexually abused children show many more psychiatric symptoms than children who have not been abused. Abuse leads to fear, PTSD, behavioral problems, contravention, the presence of incompatible sexual behavior with age, anxiety, and depression (Kendall-Tackett, Williams, and Finkelhor 1993).

Attachment theory suggests that a child's adaptation is closely linked to his or her relationships with caregivers from whom the child successfully or unsuccessfully receives emotional and physical support (Bowlby 2008). When children experience many victimizations, the developmental and security needs of the children are unable to be met by caregivers. Adolescents who have experienced more than one victimization present with more social anxiety, a decreased trust in others, and more social alienation than adolescents with one or no victimization.

Difficulties, which include impairment in the relational and therapeutic structures required for successful treatment results in establishing relationships, desensitize triggers and developing skills and have been observed in adolescents who have experienced a large number of victimizations (Cohen, Mannarino, and Deblinger 2016; Cohen et al. 2012; Kerr, Stattin, and Trost 1999).

A study comparing three groups of women - those who were sexually abused in both childhood and adulthood, those who were sexually abused only in adulthood, and those who never experienced sexual abuse - showed that the rates of PTSD were not only high but also equivalent in both the groups who were abused. There were also higher rates of alexithymia, dissociative disorder, and suicide attempts in the women who faced revictimization. Additionally, women who went through revictimization have shown that they have significant interpersonal problems. Evidence has shown that some of the problems related to affect regulation, such as alexithymia and dissociation, are risk factors for sexual assault. In addition, affect dysregulations such as emotional flooding and numbing have been shown to be risk factors for alcohol and drug use and are often reported as coping mechanisms that aim to reduce the dolorous effects of trauma. This, too, has also been shown to be a risk factor for sexual assault (Cloitre and Rosenberg 2006; Cloitre, Scarvalone, and Difede 1997).

In the results of a study about at what point a man might have gone "too far" (female university students were asked to listen to a date sketch that progressed from "verbal insistence to forcing" and to push the stop button when the man went too far), it was determined that women who experienced revictimization pressed the button later than those who never experienced victimization or experienced it only once (Van Wie, Gross, and Marx 1995).

Interpersonal Schemas

Our views, patterns, and schemas of ourselves and others are determined in childhood. The desire of children to engage with eligible caregivers is biological. They are dependent on elders for basic needs such as protection and nourishment (Bowlby 1969). In the context of the developmental model of interpersonal schemas, in a study examining women with a history of sexual abuse in childhood and women who endured revictimization, women victims of incest think that their kinspeople (mother, father, friend) will behave imperiously and keep their distance. However, women who have never been abused expect loving and respectful reactions to their independence from their relatives (Cloitre, Cohen, and Scarvalone 2002).

It can be assumed that affect dysregulation can trigger attachment dysregulation and that attachment dysregulation can also trigger affect dysregulation. After all, both situations will foster each other. When people's interpersonal schemas are formed in a negative way, they are often put in open, suitable, or vulnerable situations, which could include violence.

ADULTHOOD

It has been revealed that guilt and shame are embedded in the phenomenology of trauma victims. Guilt and shame lead to the tendency for the survivors to be under the yoke of trauma because they convince themselves that they played an important role in the occurrence of a tragic and irreparable outcome. They also tend to conclude that the result reflects their entire individuality, personality, or character (Kubany and Watson 2003). In a study of 212 physically and/or sexually abused women diagnosed with PTSD, it was established that 75 percent of them reported a feeling of guilt that was associated with a medium or higher level of abuse. Studies have shown that the feeling of guilt that is connected with trauma is a common problem among war veterans, victims of physical and sexual abuse, and those connected with technological disasters, accidents, suicides, murders, sudden illness, and surviving family members (Kubany et al. 1995; Kubany and Ralston 1998). A study of 548 female college students determined that shame mediated the relationship between sexual abuse in childhood and adult victimization. The results also showed that survivors from sexual abuse in childhood with higher levels of shame were more likely to go through revictimization than both nonabused women and abused women with low levels of internalized shame (Kessler and Bieschke 1999). In a study of 157 victims, evaluations were made immediately after the trauma, and in the sixth month, it was found that the feelings of shame and anger detected at the first stage were the only independent predictors of PTSD symptoms in the first month among all variables. The feeling of shame itself was found to be the predictor of PTSD, which was diagnosed six months later. The most common cause of embarrassment among participants with high a level of shame was that they did not take adequate measures to prevent victimization or trauma (Andrews et al. 2000).

It should not be overlooked that feelings of guilt and shame can be experienced by epigenetic, prenatal, and childhood psychosomatization transfers. A fault or crime committed in the previous generation or in one's own life, the consciousness of surviving when others were killed, the witnessing of violence and not being able to save the victim subjected to violence, dereliction, and a situation in which one is underrated or experiences a sense of worthlessness can easily activate feelings of guilt and shame. Feelings of dereliction and worthlessness can also come from taking care of another sibling and being sick of the mother, divorce, having to work in a remote place where the father once worked, and the death of a caregiver. Those who feel worthless or guilty may have direct motivation to punish themselves, or they may react to those who put themselves in the situation. However, they often direct their aggression toward themselves since their physicality or self-confidence is not enough to fend off the aggression of others.

CONCLUSION

It has been observed that those who have been subjected to various acts of violence are not attacked due to physical weakness but are victimized by epigenetics, the state of the pregnancy of their mother, and the burdens of childhood, adolescence, and adulthood because not everyone who is the victim of violence is physically weak. Since victims of violence often experience feelings of guilt and shame in their unconsciousness or consciousness, they may also develop false beliefs that they need to be punished for their guilt. These false beliefs sometimes emerge with passive-aggressive behaviors and can lead to becoming vulnerable to an attack by someone else.

In cases of violence, the characteristics of the perpetrators, the analyses of the dynamics of aggression, and treatment and support mechanisms should be prioritized. It is also important to provide treatment and rehabilitation to the victims through psychotherapy and help them with the false beliefs created by those burdens. The prevention of violence can be obtained through awareness of the victim profile and placing importance on their therapy.

REFERENCES

Andrews, B., Brewin, C. R., Rose, S., & Kirk, M. (2000). Predicting PTSD symptoms in victims of violent crime: The role of shame, anger, and childhood abuse. *Journal of Abnormal Psychology*, 109(1), 69.

Arata, C. M., & Lindman, L. (2002). Marriage, child abuse, and sexual revictimization. *Journal of Interpersonal Violence*, 17(9), 953-971.

Bender, A. (2015). *Suicide Sweeping Indian Country is Genocide*. People's World.

Bergman, K., Sarkar, P., Glover, V., & O'Connor, T. G. (2010). Maternal prenatal cortisol and infant cognitive development: Moderation by infant-mother attachment. *Biological Psychiatry*, 67(11), 1026-1032.

Bowlby, J. (1969). *Attachment: Attachment and loss*. New York: Basic.

Bowlby, J. (2008). *Attachment*. Basic books.

Burggren, W. (2016). Epigenetic inheritance and its role in evolutionary biology: re-evaluation and new perspectives. *Biology*, 5(2), 24.

Carone, B. R., Fauquier, L., Habib, N., Shea, J. M., Hart, C. E., Li, R., Zamore, P. D. (2010). Paternally induced transgenerational environmental reprogramming of metabolic gene expression in mammals. *Cell*, 143(7), 1084-1096.

Charak, R., DiLillo, D., Messman-Moore, T. L., & Gratz, K. L. (2018). Latent classes of lifetime sexual victimization characteristics in women in emerging adulthood: Differential relations with emotion dysregulation. *Psychology of Violence*, 8(5), 570.

Charak, R., Eshelman, L. R., & Messman-Moore, T. L. (2019). Latent classes of childhood maltreatment, adult sexual assault, and revictimization in men: Differences in masculinity, anger, and substance use. *Psychology of Men & Masculinities*, 20(4), 503.

Charak, R., Vang, M. L., Shevlin, M., Ben-Ezra, M., Karatzias, T., & Hyland, P. (2020). Lifetime Interpersonal Victimization Profiles and Mental Health Problems in a Nationally Representative Panel of Trauma-Exposed Adults from the United Kingdom. *Journal of Traumatic Stres*, 33(5), 654-664.

Classen, C. C., Palesh, O. G., & Aggarwal, R. (2005). Sexual revictimization: A review of the empirical literature. *Trauma, Violence, & Abuse*, 6(2), 103-129.

Clemmons, J. C., DiLillo, D., Martinez, I. G., DeGue, S., & Jeffcott, M. (2003). Co-occurring forms of child maltreatment and adult adjustment reported by Latina college students. *Child Abuse & Neglect*, 27(7), 751-767.

Cloitre, M., Cohen, L. R., & Scarvalone, P. (2002). Understanding revictimization among childhood sexual abuse survivors: An interpersonal schema approach. *Journal of Cognitive Psychotherapy*, 16(1), 91.

Cloitre, M., & Rosenberg, A. (2006). Sexual revictimization. *Cognitive-Behavioral Therapies for Trauma*, 321-361.

Cloitre, M., Scarvalone, P., & Difede, J. (1997). Posttraumatic stress disorder, self-and interpersonal dysfunction among sexually retraumatized women. *Journal of Traumatic Stress*, 10(3), 437-452.

Cloitre, M., Tardiff, K., Marzuk, P. M., Leon, A. C., & Portera, L. (1996). Childhood abuse and subsequent sexual assault among female inpatients. *Journal of Traumatic Stress*, 9(3), 473-482.

Cohen, J. A., Mannarino, A. P., & Deblinger, E. (2016). *Treating trauma and traumatic grief in children and adolescents*. Guilford Publications.

Cohen, J. A., Mannarino, A. P., Kliethermes, M., & Murray, L. A. (2012). Trauma-focused CBT for youth with complex trauma. *Child Abuse & Neglect*, 36(6), 528-541.

Dias, B. G., & Ressler, K. J. (2014). Parental olfactory experience influences behavior and neural structure in subsequent generations. *Nature Neuroscience*, 17(1), 89-96.

Erickson, M. F., Egeland, B., & Pianta, R. (1989). The effects of maltreatment on the development of young children.

Fergusson, D. M., Horwood, L. J., & Lynskey, M. T. (1997). Childhood sexual abuse, adolescent sexual behaviors and sexual revictimization. *Child Abuse & Neglect*, 21(8), 789-803.

Finegersh, A., & Homanics, G. E. (2014). Paternal alcohol exposure reduces alcohol drinking and increases behavioral sensitivity to alcohol selectively in male offspring. *PloS One*, 9(6), e99078.

Glausiusz, J. (2014). *Searching chromosomes for the legacy of trauma.* Nature News.

Hennessy, K. D., Rabideau, G. J., Cicchetti, D., & Cummings, E. M. (1994). Responses of physically abused and nonabused children to different forms of interadult anger. *Child Development*, 65(3), 815-828.

Howes, C., & Eldredge, R. (1985). Responses of abused, neglected, and non-maltreated children to the behaviors of their peers. *Journal of Applied Developmental Psychology*, 6(2-3), 261-270.

Hughes, V. (2014). Sperm RNA carries marks of trauma. *Nature*, 508(7496), 296-297.

Irwin, H. J. (1999). Violent and nonviolent revictimization of women abused in childhood. *Journal of Interpersonal Violence*, 14(10), 1095-1110.

Jankowski, M. K., Leitenberg, H., Henning, K., & Coffey, P. (2002). Parental caring as a possible buffer against sexual revictimization in young adult survivors of child sexual abuse. *Journal of Traumatic Stress: Official Publication of the International Society for Traumatic Stress Studies*, 15(3), 235-244.

Kendall-Tackett, K. A., Williams, L. M., & Finkelhor, D. (1993). Impact of sexual abuse on children: a review and synthesis of recent empirical studies. *Psychological Bulletin*, 113(1), 164.

Kerr, M., Stattin, H., & Trost, K. (1999). To know you is to trust you: Parents' trust is rooted in child disclosure of information. *Journal of Adolescence*, 22(6), 737-752.

Kessler, B. L., & Bieschke, K. J. (1999). A retrospective analysis of shame, dissociation, and adult victimization in survivors of childhood sexual abuse. *Journal of Counseling Psychology*, 46(3), 335.

Kubany, E. S., Abueg, F. R., Owens, J. A., Brennan, J. M., Kaplan, A. S., & Watson, S. B. (1995). Initial examination of a multidimensional model of trauma-related guilt: Applications to combat veterans and battered women. *Journal of Psychopathology and Behavioral Assessment*, 17(4), 353-376.

Kubany, E. S., & Ralston, T. C. (1998). Cognitive therapy for trauma-related guilt. *Cognitive-Behavioral Therapies for Trauma*, 124-161.

Kubany, E. S., & Watson, S. B. (2003). Guilt: Elaboration of a multidimensional model. *Psychological Record*, 53(1), 51-90.

Lambrot, R., Xu, C., Saint-Phar, S., Chountalos, G., Cohen, T., Paquet, M., Kimmins, S. (2013). Low paternal dietary folate alters the mouse sperm epigenome and is associated with negative pregnancy outcomes. *Nature Communications*, 4, 2889.

Merrill, L. L., Newell, C. E., Thomsen, C. J., Gold, S. R., Milner, J. S., Koss, M. P., & Rosswork, S. G. (1999). Childhood abuse and sexual revictimization in a female Navy recruit sample. *Journal of Traumatic Stress: Official Publication of the International Society for Traumatic Stress Studies*, 12(2), 211-225.

Messman-Moore, T. L., & Long, P. J. (2003). The role of childhood sexual abuse sequelae in the sexual revictimization of women: An empirical review and theoretical reformulation. *Clinical Psychology Review*, 23(4), 537-571.

Nestler, E. J. (2014). Epigenetic mechanisms of depression. *JAMA Psychiatry*, 71(4), 454-456.

Pembrey, M. E., Bygren, L. O., Kaati, G., Edvinsson, S., Northstone, K., Sjöström, M., & Golding, J. (2006). Sex-specific, male-line transgenerational responses in humans. *European Journal of Human Genetics*, 14(2), 159-166.

Roodman, A. A., & Clum, G. A. (2001). Revictimization rates and method variance: A meta-analysis. *Clinical Psychology Review*, 21(2), 183-204.

Rouse, A. (2015). Holocaust survivors pass the genetic damage of their trauma on to their children, researchers find. *Mail Online*, 21.

Sack, D. (2014). When Emotional Trauma is a Family Affair. *Psychology Today*.

Sanders, B., & Moore, D. L. (1999). Childhood maltreatment and date rape. *Journal of Interpersonal Violence*, 14(2), 115-124.

Schaaf, K. K., & McCanne, T. R. (1998). Relationship of childhood sexual, physical, and combined sexual and physical abuse to adult victimization and posttraumatic stress disorder. *Child Abuse & Neglect*, 22(11), 1119-1133.

Shields, A., & Cicchetti, D. (1998). Reactive aggression among maltreated children: The contributions of attention and emotion dysregulation. *Journal of Clinical Child Psychology*, 27(4), 381-395.

Shields, A. M., Cicchetti, D., & Ryan, R. M. (1994). The development of emotional and behavioral self-regulation and social competence among maltreated school-age children. *Development and Psychopathology*, 6, 57-57.

Vaissière, T., Sawan, C., & Herceg, Z. (2008). Epigenetic interplay between histone modifications and DNA methylation in gene silencing. *Mutation Research/Reviews in Mutation Research*, 659(1-2), 40-48.

Van Wie, V. E., Gross, A. M., & Marx, B. P. (1995). Females' perception of date rape: An examination of two contextual variables. *Violence against Women*, 1(4), 351-365.

Weintraub, P., & Verny, T. (2014). *Nurturing the unborn child: A nine-month program for soothing, stimulating, and communicating with your baby*. Open Road Media.

Widom, C. S., Czaja, S. J., & Dutton, M. A. (2008). Childhood victimization and lifetime revictimization. *Child Abuse & Neglect*, 32(8), 785-796.

Wyatt, G. E., Guthrie, D., & Notgrass, C. M. (1992). Differential effects of women's child sexual abuse and subsequent sexual revictimization. *Journal of Consulting and Clinical Psychology*, 60(2), 167.

Yao, Y., Robinson, A. M., Zucchi, F. C., Robbins, J. C., Babenko, O., Kovalchuk, O., Metz, G. A. (2014). Ancestral exposure to stress epigenetically programs preterm birth risk and adverse maternal and newborn outcomes. *BMC Medicine*, 12(1), 121.

Yehuda, R., & Seckl, J. (2011). Minireview: stress-related psychiatric disorders with low cortisol levels: a metabolic hypothesis. *Endocrinology*, 152(12), 4496-4503.

In: Forensic Psychiatry …
Editor: Nursen Turan Yurtsever
ISBN: 978-1-53619-530-9

Chapter 5

Massive Traumatic Events and Posttraumatic Stress Disorder

Mesut Yıldız *
Department of Psychiatry, Marmara University,
School of Medicine, Istanbul, Turkey

Abstract

Posttraumatic stress disorder (PTSD) is a psychiatric disorder that may occur in people who have experienced or witnessed a traumatic event such as a natural disaster, a serious accident, a terrorist act, war/combat, or rape or who have been threatened with death, sexual violence, or serious injury. Individuals with PTSD may have impairments in aspects of their psychological, physical, interpersonal, and occupational lives. PTSD usually has a chronic course and causes disruptions in the general and social functioning of the person. PTSD can be both underdiagnosed and overdiagnosed in clinical settings. There are clear differences in the clinical approach to PTSD cases and the forensic perspective. The medicolegal approach is different from the clinical viewpoint. Psychiatrists are frequently asked for evaluations of traumatic events in civil and criminal matters. Psychiatrists are asked to evaluate if the traumatic event caused or

* Corresponding Author's E-mail: mesut.yildiz@marmara.edu.tr.

contributed to a psychiatric disorder or a functional impairment. They are also asked to make a distinction between causal and contributing factors. In addition, the factors that contribute to the person's current mental state and functionality should be well reviewed, and a possible malingering should not be overlooked. This chapter will review the clinical and ethical implications in evaluating patients with PTSD in a forensic setting.

INTRODUCTION

Posttraumatic stress disorder (PTSD) is a disorder characterized by the reexperiencing or avoidance of symptoms after a life-threatening event and the possible accompaniment of alterations in mood and cognition and hyperarousal symptoms (APA 2013).

The prevalence of traumatic experiences is remarkable high among all populations. The World Mental Health Survey Consortium reports that 70 percent of the world's population has reported exposure to a traumatic event (Benjet 2016). Although traumatic experiences are frequent, the prevalence of PTSD is relatively low. Not all people exposed to trauma develop PTSD or need psychiatric treatment. The lifetime prevalence of PTSD is 3.9 percent overall and 5.6 percent among respondents exposed to trauma (Benjet 2016). According to the National Comorbidity Survey, even though 61 percent of men and 51 percent of women have been exposed to a traumatic experience at some point in their lives, the lifetime prevalence of PTSD is 8 percent and 20 percent, respectively (Kessler 1995). Most patients get better without psychiatric intervention because of their coping abilities and the help they receive through their social environment. On the other hand, some may need psychiatric or psychological help to move on and get better.

Individuals with a mental disorder have higher rates of trauma-related disorders compared with the general population (Mauritz 2013). It is likely that in settings where forensic assessment is conducted, there are relatively more people who have experienced traumatic experiences in their lifetimes (Rocchio 2020). These data show that trauma histories are quite common in psychiatric practice. In addition, trauma stories are frequently encountered in forensic psychiatry evaluations. One thing to note is that PTSD patients are reluctant to talk about their trauma. This can sometimes make it difficult to detect PTSD.

The validity and reliability of the diagnosis of PTSD have been questioned due to issues such as financial benefit expectations of persons affiliated with PTSD and avoidance of criminal cases, and its acceptance by diagnostic systems has been delayed (Pitman 1996). After the acceptance of the diagnosis of PTSD, it has become important to realize that a mental impairment and loss of functionality may occur in a person due to stressful situations. It has come to the forefront that mental distress may develop in cases of physical damage, and this mental distress may also be a subject of compensation.

Psychiatrists are frequently asked for an evaluation of traumatic events in civil and criminal matters. In terms of a forensic evaluation, psychiatrists are asked to assess the impact of traumatic events and express their opinion about the traumatic event's connection to some psycholegal issues (Rocchio 2020). Psychiatrists are usually asked to prepare a formal report and/or provide testimony about their evaluations. Evaluators may be asked to evaluate the functional level of the person before and after the traumatic event, whether there were other traumatic events that could affect the person's mental state before the mentioned traumatic event, and the mental status of the person before and after the traumatic event (Foote and Lareau 2013). In addition, evaluators can also assist the court as expert witnesses by presenting scientific data on PTSD in cases while also writing and presenting their opinion. Besides, psychiatrists may be asked to assess the impact of traumatic event(s) on the individual's state of mind at the time a crime occurred or explain the behavior during orafter an alleged criminal act. They may also be asked to give their opinion whether the presence of a traumatic event will be a reason for mitigation in criminal cases. Psychiatrists should be able to prepare a scientifically based, consistent, and persuasive report by taking into account both psychiatry and law. In doing all these, it is essential that psychiatrists act in accordance with ethical principles. They should take into account the international medical ethical rules, the guidelines of professional organizations, and scientific and professional information.

In fact, most psychiatrists have a clinical understanding of how PTSD is diagnosed and its treatment options. The main difficulty lies in the forensic assessment of people with possible PTSD. Understanding the distinction between clinical and forensic roles is of critical importance at this point (Greenberg 1997). There are marked differences between a treating clinician and a forensic psychiatrist in terms of their mission, method, and ethical duty. The mission of the treating clinician is the alleviation of emotional suffering of the patients. On the other hand, the forensic psychiatrist searches for relative objective data to determine an accurate diagnosis, recommends treatment, and gives opinions about prognosis and causal factors. While the clinician focuses more on what the patient says about his or her experience, the forensic psychiatrist reviews all available data, including all medical and legal records and psychological testing when needed. While the clinician takes the approach toward acting for the benefit of the patient, the forensic psychiatrist tries to reach the truth in light of the available data (Fox and Levy 2013). The psychiatrist, as a clinician, has little interest in the law, and generally, most of the information the clinician receives is from the patient and he or she is not informed about any possible fabricated information. These limitations sometimes present difficulties when there is a psycholegal situation. Moreover, there can be an increase in role confusion and ethical problems when a clinician is asked legal questions about his or her patient (Greenberg 1997).

In terms of forensic medicine, there are diverse points about PTSD that should be considered. It is important to know whether the person has had any psychiatric disorder before the traumatic event, the course of this psychiatric disorder, and its effect on the functionality of the person. Whether the trauma has caused a new mental disorder in the person or whether it has caused an exacerbation in the preexisting mental disorder should also be considered. In addition, the factors that contribute to the person's current mental state and functionality should be well reviewed, and a possible malingering should not be overlooked (Jovanovic 2016).

HISTORY TAKING: MATTERS TO BE CONSIDERED

According to the Diagnostic and Statistical Manual of Mental Disorders, Fifth Edition (DSM-5), PTSD diagnosis requires exposure to a traumatic eventin criterion A. The DSM-5 definition of trauma requires "actual or threatened death, serious injury, or sexual violence." Not all stressful events fall within the definition of trauma. DSM-IV-TR defined trauma as "threat to physical integrity,"but this definition was changed in DSM-5 (APA 2000). Stressful life events and illnesses such as job loss, divorce, terminal cancer, and heart attack are not considered trauma according to DSM-5. Clinicians should be careful when making a diagnosis.

If the clinician is faced with a case file, then it should be clarified whether the incident falls within the definition of a traumatic event by collecting data from as many sources as possible (witness statements of the incident, documents in the case file, accident reports, medical reports, epicrisis, etc.). In particular, if there is uncertainty about the documentation of traumas of the past years, then it should be stated in the forensic report as is.

Since people can easily access information about PTSD and diagnostic criteria from many sources, they can give a history if they have typical symptoms. Thus, it is generally advised to make a nondirective interview first and ask the key questions and use semi-structured scales afterwards. This approach will provide a better understanding of the person's own experience and make it easier to prevent the person from falsifying his or her symptoms (Jovanovic 2016).

Using semi-structured interview scales like the Clinician-Administered PTSD Scale (CAPS) isuseful in taking histories of people with possible PTSD. An advantage of these semi-structured scales is that the detailed data obtained here allow a comparative assessment of the individual's history, case file, medical reports, etc. In order to distinguish genuine PTSD from malingering or factitious PTSD, the semi-structured interviews give a multitude of information. Some clinicians note that individuals who genuinely suffer from PTSD describe a wide variety of symptoms when describing events, but individuals feigning or exaggerating their symptoms focus on specific symptoms (Jovanovic 2016). For patients who are suspected of mitigating the symptoms of PTSD, it will be helpful for the clinician to use scales such as theStructured Inventory of Malingered Symptomatology (SIMS) or the Miller-Forensic Assessment of Symptoms (M-FAST) (Smith and Burger 2003; Miller 2005). Both scales are screening scales, and higher scores in these scales suggest further evaluation. Clinicians should also use the Minnesota Multiphasic Personality Inventory-2 (MMPI-2) todetect malingering. More than 90 percent of subjects attempting to malinger PTSD were correctly identified using the F and PK scales (Guriel 2003).

Diagnostic criterion B of PTSD requires the presence of intrusion symptoms that are associated with the traumatic event beginning after the traumatic event. Repetitive and distressing dreams and flashbacks are distinguishing features of PTSD. The emotions experienced in nightmares are generally representative of the emotions experienced during the trauma. PTSD nightmares are often purely visual and almost always accompanied by either sudden awakenings or notable body movement during sleep, a fact that should be apparent to bedmates. Although individuals experiencing flashbacks reexperience perceptual and emotional details, these flashbacks are more likely to include auditory and olfactory components. Individuals feigning PTSD generally only report the perceptual and emotional details of the trauma (Matto 2019).

It has been shown that those who imitate PTSD are generally good at imitating dreams and flashbacks but are not so good at imitating avoidance. Some people may underreport some of their symptoms or describe them incompletely. It should be evaluated whether this is due to the person's cultural background or military origin because it is known that there is sometimes underreporting in cases of malingering (Matto 2019).

Malingering of PTSD

How often is PTSD feigned? It is estimated to be around 15.7 percentand 7.4 percent in forensic and non-forensic evaluations, respectively (Rogers

1994). There may be some conscious and unconscious reasons why patients feign a diagnosis of PTSD, including to stay away from certain duties in business (avoiding military duty, avoiding work) and family life and to gain the compassion of family members; to benefit from a financial gain (obtaining a disability report or retiring with disability); to obtain drugs (such as benzodiazepines) from physicians; to receive inpatient treatment in the psychiatric ward; or to avoid or reduce criminal liability. This feigning condition is called malingering but is not considered a mental illness in DSM-5. Malingering is the fabrication or exaggeration of physical or psychological symptoms in order to achieve gain, which may include avoiding responsibility, gaining a financial compensation, or evading criminal prosecution. It can be seen in a pure or partial form. Pure malingering is not common in individuals with PTSD but involves frequent exaggeration of symptoms. Although malingering was excluded from the index in DSM-5, it receives a V code as one of the other conditions that may be a focus of clinical attention, and the criteria for when to consider malingering remains unchanged. Malingering is frequently found in association with antisocial personality disorder and to a lesser extent with histrionic personality disorder (Sequeira 2018; Lanska 2018).

Clinicians should be suspicious of malingering in cases sent in a medicolegal context if the mental distress described by the person is inconsistent with the data obtained from other sources/medical reports, if the person has had antisocial behaviors in the past, and if the person's cooperation is weak during the assessment. In some compensation cases, individuals are referred to a doctor by their legal representatives before the case to ensure that the case is turned in their favor or to increase the compensation they will receive. Therefore, the person should be asked how he or she applied for the first application and what kind of help he or she wanted. In these cases, it is typical for the person to be directed to a doctor before the case but after an accident or similar situation and to request a report from the doctor.

Occasionally, judges ask the clinician's opinion in regard to the memories of an individual and whether they are reliable and whether they can trust the individual's statements.

It is not easy for the clinician to answer these questions. However, some clinical questions will arise in regard to this topic. Are traumatic memories constant? How reliable are they? While such questions do not make much sense in the treatment of a PTSD patient by a clinician, these questions are important in a forensic situation. Studies have shown that the memories of events experienced by a person can change over time (Morgan 2005). Moreover, since it is known that memory can be impaired in stressful situations, care should be taken in this regard. In addition, it was thought that it would be better for clinicians not to comment on this issue since there is no test that measures the accuracy of traumatic memories experienced by people.

In some of the forensic cases referred for PTSD, the person had other traumas before the subject traumatic event. In this case, the clinician should consider each traumatic event separately and reveal the degree and deterioration of all of them. In addition, there is a higher possibility of reaching a more accurate result when stories are taken from people who know the situation of the person before and after the traumatic events.

In some criminal cases, it may also be that PTSD cases were submitted by judges for an assessment of the person's medical condition. Judges may consider a reduction in a person's punishment by taking into account whether the person has a psychiatric disorder, the degree, if any, and whether treatment is required.

MISATTRIBUTED PTSD DIAGNOSIS

In some cases, the symptoms attributed to PTSD may be associated with another psychiatric or medical disorder. Clinicians should rule out other psychiatric disorderssuch as depression, substance abuse, anxiety disorders, and trauma (post-concussive syndrome) that can mimic PTSD symptoms. In other words, if the suspected PTSD symptoms are associated with another medical/psychiatric disorder, it is then called misattributed PTSD. Even if the diagnosis of PTSD is clear, cases should be screened in terms of comorbid medical and psychiatric disorders. Comorbidity is quite common in PTSD—it has been shown that 92 percent of participants with PTSD have a comorbid psychiatric disorder (Brown 2001). Thus, it is important to evaluate comorbid mental disorders in cases where the criminal and legal liability of PTSD cases is evaluated or a decision is made about disability, because comorbid disorders can significantly affect the decision (Matto 2019).

Factitious PTSD

There is also another form of PTSD that is rarely discussed: factitious PTSD. If the person is intentionally fabricating PSTD symptoms in the absence of external gain, a diagnosis of factitious PTSD should be considered. Patients may fabricate these symptoms to gain the potential benefits of being in the sick role in the community. It has been observed that these people generally have expectations such as acceptance, admiration, and appreciation from their surroundings and the society they live in.

Reactivation of PTSD

DSM-5 specified a "delayed expression" of PTSD. If the full diagnostic criteria are not met until at least six months after the event, it is labeled a delayed expression of PTSD. Clinicians should be aware of this clinical phenomenon. Another clinical point to consider is that residual PTSD symptoms are generally predictors of future reactivation. Besides, it is also known that memories of a traumatic experience can be revived in a stressful situation later in life (Kinzie et al. 2002). Some authors in the field of PTSD do not accept delayed or reactivated PTSD as a true PTSD for reasons such as false attribution, exaggeration, or falsification or for people with previous medical problems applying for secondary earnings. (Sparr and Pankratz 1983; Boe et al. 2010).

Complex Trauma and Dissociation

The term complex trauma was developed to describe the symptoms following severe and repeated trauma, especially during childhood (Cook 2003). Complex trauma during early periods of life increases the risk of further traumas and victimization (Briere 2016). It has been shown that complex trauma affects a person's attention, emotions, and physical symptoms. In addition, due to the complex trauma, the person's perception of self, others, and the world is also affected (Courtois and Ford 2013; Bailey-Brand 2017). The aforementioned clinical picture seen in adults who were severely and repeatedly traumatized during their childhood is called complex posttraumatic stress disorder (cPTSD). Dissociation is especially important here. It has been reported that dissociative symptoms are more intense and more frequent in individuals with cPTSD (Hyland 2019). Dissociation regarding a traumatic event is frequently reported by offenders presenting for a forensic psychiatric examination. Presence of dissociation can be important in legal situations because it can affect judgment, criminal responsibility, and perception capacity (Paris 2019). Whether dissociation has an impact on an individual's criminal responsibility requires a detailed and sometimes difficult process for the evaluator. The evaluator should assess all the available information from the individual and collateral resources (family, friends, school, work, psychological tests, medical records, forensic reports, etc.) and court. When taking history from the relatives of these individuals, it is important to keep in mind that the person giving the story may also be responsible for the traumatic event (Rocchio 2020).

The individual's personality, prior psychiatric history, substance use, and prior history of dissociative events should be carefully studied and learned. The individual's state of mind before and near the time of the crime should also be obtained to make a comprehensive evaluation (Bourget 2017). For a patient exposed to trauma, it is particularly important that all findings occurring after trauma in the case are detected and documented to prevent the loss of rights and for the legal process to proceed in a healthy manner (Can 2013; Şener 2014).

PTSD as a Mitigating Factor

If it is thought that the mental state of the offender during the crime he or she committed influenced the formation of the crime, then his or her mental disorder can be considered as a mitigating factor (Berger 2012). In cases in which PTSD is thought to have a role in an offense, if the person's response is disproportionate to the provocative event or if the circumstances reevoked the original traumatic event, then PTSD could be evaluated as a mitigating factor in sentencing.

Ethical Considerations

In the forensic evaluation of cases of people with PTSD, there are risks for the clinician and trauma survivor that include vicarious trauma and re-traumatization (Sharon L Mailloux 2013). The revisiting and processing of traumatic memories increases the risk of re-traumatization. Recalling or discussing traumatic memories may create autobiographical landmarks, which can have important effects on the individual's sense of identity (Bernsten 2005). Sometimes, the individual being evaluated for possible PTSD may also have traumatic events prior to the alleged trauma. In this case, clinicians may be asked to evaluate the impact of prior traumas and sequelae of these traumas on the individual's life.

It is important for psychiatrists to stay away from multiple roles. If psychiatrists are not able to use their knowledge effectively and objectively due to some interest between them and the evaluee, they should not assume a professional role (Yadav 2017).

The competence of the clinician, his or her knowledge in the field, and his or her attention to ethical issues are important issues in regard to re-traumatization of the PTSD survivor (Sharon L Mailloux 2013). In terms of ethics, the mental health practitioner should first question whether the issues to be evaluated are related to his or her area of expertise and whether it is appropriate for him or her to evaluate the case (Brand 2016). The psychiatrist should not provide opinions for which he or she does not have sufficient basis and should consult other professionals and look for scientific literature where needed. When ethical conflicts arise, the psychiatrist should not hesitate to consult the ethics committee of his or her institution when necessary.

Objectivity is important when assessing individuals in a forensic environment. For the solution of a forensic psychiatric problem, it is essential to assess the individual in a broad bio-psycho-social dimension and examine the problem within the framework of ethical principles and laws with an objective judgment without prejudice in this spectrum. An empathic approach is important in therapeutic settings in psychiatry, but when evaluating forensic cases, this approach can have some disadvantages. Empathy should not be used as a therapeutic technique because it can cause the psychiatrist to forget the purpose of the evaluation process (Shuman 2010).

Although a fully objective approach is not always possible, it is important to take care that the empathic approach does not affect professional views and approaches when evaluating forensic cases (Gold 2004; Shuman 2010). The forensic psychiatrist should also be careful about others' opinions and instructions that may lead to false information and opinions about the case (Fox and Levy 2013).

Trauma survivors need to feel safe and in control. Often, they want to express their emotions and know about the procedure and what comes next. An appropriate explanation of how the process will proceed will ease the interview environment. Protecting the confidentiality of the person is one of the primary duties of the psychiatrist, and precautions should be taken in this regard. It should also be known that this confidentiality has its limits. The disclosure must be made only with the client's consent or consent of the legally authorized individual; it can also be made without the client's consent only if mandated by law or when the psychologist uses the information for consultation or protection of the client (APA 2010). The psychiatrist should be clear about the rules and expectations. Boundary crossings and unacceptable conduct should not be allowed.

From an ethical perspective, the evaluator should be familiar with the judicial and administrative rules (APA 2017). In a legal situation, the person making the assessment should have a different point of view, understand the underlying meaning of the law, and have basic knowledge of law and forensic medicine (Cantürk 2012).

When evaluating a traumatized person in a forensic setting, the evaluator should consider the traumatized person's age, gender, race, ethnicity, culture, religion, disability, language, and socioeconomical status (APA 2017). The evaluator should also pay attention to how the person's cultural background defines this trauma as well as the impact of their culture on their posttraumatic experiences.

An insufficient clinician may ask deep and hasty questions too quickly with good intentions to understand and help. At times, stories told by PTSD patients may be so interesting that the clinician may try to satiate his or her curiosity. In an effort to quickly understand or pay attention to the story rather than the individual with PTSD, an evaluator may cause more harm than good to the individual (Campesino 2007). Before asking questions about the traumatic event, the clinician should first establish a therapeutic relationship with the individual and then look at the individual's perspectives, beliefs and values, and life experiences before the traumatic event. These may help the clinician better understand the trauma from the individual's perspective (Brown 2008). When talking to traumatized people about their trauma, it is important to interview them in a respectful and culturally appropriate manner (Goldsmith 2004).

In addition, inexperienced clinicians may also be neglectful and ignore or minimize the trauma. The exhausting nature of the work can also result in carelessness by the inexperienced clinician. This attitude may emotionally re-traumatize the PTSD survivor (Tjeltveit 2010). Since re-traumatization is associated with increased mental health problems, drug/alcohol addictions, and violence toward other people, clinicians should be careful when taking histories from these individuals (Covington 2012).

RECORD KEEPING AND REPORT WRITING

Copies of all sources such as the information obtained, the interviews made, the tests performed, and the medical reports should be kept properly. It's important to be clear about how records will be kept and who will have access to them. When a person comes for an evaluation, it should first be mentioned who will have access to the information and how that information will be communicated.

Since the forensic assessment often needs to be completed in a short time, the evaluator should keep in mind that this period can be tiring and degrading for the trauma victim and breaks should be given where necessary. While writing the report, a scientific evaluation should be made in light of existing findings, data, and testing; the evaluator should not comment outside of the available data (Brand and Schielke 2017).

The level of detail to be included in the written document should be well evaluated. Unnecessary information that will not be involved in decision-making should not be included in the records or written report. Consultation with other professionals may be useful, and the psychiatrist should be careful when writing details of the case when consulting with other professionals. The psychiatrist should also be familiar with the similarities and differences between the various disciplines' approaches and ethical perceptions. This will help guide conversations and help others understand the differences between other branches of medicine.

For illustrative purposes, two case reports will be presented here.

Case 1

A twenty-year-old male patient came in for an evaluation of suitability for military service and had symptoms of PTSD, which he stated developed after a traffic accident. It was observed that there was an inconsistency between his clinical symptoms and mental state examination. His past medical records were requested, and an MMPI test was requested for psychological evaluation. The MMPI test was found to be invalid. It was understood from his medical records that he had been followed up with different diagnoses such as depression, anxiety disorder, and atypical psychotic disorder from different hospitals. It was understood from his follow-up stories that he had prominent antisocial personality traits and manipulative actions. This case is an example that shows that we should not make hasty decisions while making decisions on the facts and that we should not avoid requesting additional resources and psychological tests when necessary.

Case 2

A thirty-two-year-old military personnel applied to an outpatient clinic for a disability report. He was talking about lack of sleep, flashbacks, and nightmares that had developed after a gunfight in his mission about four years ago. From time to time, he had contractions in his body, and he was exhibiting aggressive behaviors (hitting objects, walls). These aggressive behaviors were so severe that there were injuries in different parts of his body. He stated that when he thought of the traumatic event he had experienced in the past, he had contractions in his body that caused him to harm the environment and himself. He stated that his personal and social functionality was restricted due to these symptoms. He used many different antidepressants in the past and stated that he did not benefit from any of them. He was admitted to the in-patient clinic for a detailed observation and evaluation. In the first days, he had conversion-like symptoms and intermittent agitated behavior. These symptoms decreased within weeks, and his communication with other patients increased. In the detailed story, he talked about his difficulties with his profession, and over time it became clear that he had an expectation about disability. This person suffered a trauma, but it turned out that he exaggerated his symptoms in anticipation of disability. The clinical significance of this case is that it is easier to make a decision when information and observations increase when the cases are followed up several times or when necessary and when clinicians are not sure about the diagnosis.

Conclusion

Traumatic events do not cause the same emotional response or injury to all persons who experience a traumatic event. Although PTSD cases are easy to diagnose clinically, there are certain difficulties when faced in forensic situations. Therefore, in the evaluation of cases with PTSD, it is helpful to follow a standard methodological approach and conduct interviews with the individual by obtaining information, excluding medical and psychiatric conditions that may cause confusion, from collateral and related sources, evaluating whether symptoms are feigned or exaggerated, and using psychological tests when necessary. Psychiatrists are asked to evaluate if the traumatic event caused or contributed to a psychiatric disorder or functional impairment. They are also asked to make a distinction between causal and contributing factors. In addition, the factors that contribute to the person's current mental state and functionality should be well reviewed, and a possible malingering should not be overlooked. Given the subjective nature of PTSD, false attribution and exaggeration, and falsification of data and secondary gains, the forensic psychiatrist should be careful when evaluating cases with PTSD.

References

American Psychiatric Association (2000). *Diagnostic and statistical manual of mental disorders* (4th ed., Text Revision). Washington, DC: Author.

American Psychiatric Association: *Diagnostic and Statistical Manual of Mental Disorders*, Fifth Edition. Washington, DC: American Psychiatric Association, 2013.

American Psychological Association (2010) Ethical principles of psychologists and code of conduct. *Am Psychol* 65.

American Psychological Association. (2017). *Ethical principles of psychologists and code of conduct.*

Bailey, T. D., and Brand, B. L. (2017). Traumatic dissociation: Theory, research, and treatment. *Clinical Psychology: Science and Practice*, 24(2), 170–185.

Benjet, C., Bromet, E., Karam, E. G., Kessler, R. C., McLaughlin, K. A., Ruscio, A. M., Shahly, V., Stein, D. J., Petukhova, M., Hill, E. (2016). The epidemiology of traumatic event exposure worldwide: Results from the World Mental Health Survey Consortium. *Psychological Medicine*, 46, 327–343.

Berger, O., McNiel, D. E., and Binder, R. L. (2012). PTSD as a criminal defense: a review of case law. *Journal of the American Academy of Psychiatry and the Law Online*, 40(4), 509-521.

Bernsten, D., Willert, M., & Rubin, D. C. (2005). Splintered memories or vivid landmarks? Qualities and organization of traumatic memories with and without PTSD. *Applied Cognitive Psychology*, 17, 675-693.

Boe, H. J., Holgersen, K. H., and Holen, A. (2010). Reactivation of posttraumatic stress in male disaster survivors: The role of residual symptoms. *Journal of Anxiety Disorders*, 24(4), 397-402.

Bourget, D., Gagne, P., and Wood, S. F. (2017). Dissociation: Defining the concept in criminal forensic psychiatry. *Journal of the American Academy of Psychiatry and the Law*.

Brand, B. L. (2016). The necessity of clinical training in trauma and dissociation. *Journal of Anxiety and Depression*, 5(251), 10-4172.

Brand, B. L., Schielke, H. J., and Brams, J. S. (2017). Assisting the courts in understanding and connecting with experiences of disconnection: Addressing trauma-related dissociation as a forensic psychologist, part I. *Psychological Injury and Law*, 10(4), 283–297.

Briere, J., Agee, E., and Dietrich, A. (2016). Cumulative trauma and current posttraumatic stress disorder status in general population and inmate samples. *Psychological Trauma*, 8(4), 439–446.

Brown T. A., Campbell L. A., Lehman C. L. Current and lifetime comorbidity of the DSM-IV anxiety and mood disorders in a large clinical sample. *Journal of Abnormal Psychology* 110:585–99, 2001.

Brown, L. (2008). *Cultural competence in trauma therapy: Beyond the flashback.* Washington, DC: American Psychological Association.

Campesino, M. (2007). Homicide bereavement: Reflections on the therapeutic relationship in trauma research. *Qualitative Inquiry*, 13, 541-553.

Can, İ. Ö., Uyaniker, Z. D., Ulas, H., Karabag, G., Cimilli, C., and Salacin, S. (2013). Travma Magdurlarinda Ruhsal Travma Bulgulari/Mental Findings in Trauma Victims. *Noro-Psikyatri Arsivi*, 50(3), 230.

Cantürk G. (2012). Adli psikiyatri alanında yasal düzenlemeler. *Türkiye Klinikleri J Forensic Medicine* (9):66-73.

Cook, A., Blaustein, M., Spinazzola, J., and Van der Kolk, B. (2003). Complex trauma in children and adolescents: White paper from the national child traumatic stress network complex trauma task force. *Los Angeles: National Center for Child Traumatic Stress.*

Courtois, C. A., and Ford, J. D. (2013). *Treatment of complex trauma: A sequenced, relationship-based approach.* New York: Guilford Press.

Covington, S. (2012). *Proceedings from beyond trauma: A healing journey for women.* Red Deer, Alberta, Canada: Institute for Relational Development.

Foote, W. E., and Lareau, C. R. (2013). Psychological evaluation of emotional damages in tort cases. In *Handbook of psychology: Forensic psychology* (Vol. 11, 2nd ed., pp. 172–200). Hoboken: Wiley.

Fox M. L. and Levy M. I. (2013). The Use of Forensic Psychiatry in Catastrophic Injury and Multi-Party Litigation. *Expert Evidence Report* 13 (23): 623-29.

Gold, L. (2004). *Sexual harassment: Psychiatric assessment in employment litigation.* Washington, DC: American Psychiatric Publishing.

Goldsmith, R., Barlow, M., and Freyd, J. (2004). Knowing and not knowing about trauma: Implications for therapy. *Psychotherapy: Theory, Research, Practice, Training*, 41, 448-463.

Greenberg, S. A., and Shuman, D. W. (1997). Irreconcilable conflict between therapeutic and forensic roles. *Professional Psychology: Research and Practice*, 28, 50–57.

Guriel J., Fremouw W., Assessing malingered posttraumatic stress disorder: a critical review. *Clin Psychol Review* 23:881–904, 2003.

Herman J. L. (1992) Complex PTSD – a syndrome in survivors of prolonged and repeated trauma. *Journal of Traumatic Stress*, 5: 377–91.

https://canadiem.org/wp-content/uploads/2017/10/CC.-Ep.-114-Factitious-Disorders-and-Malingering-Ch.-104-Rosens-9th-Ed.-.pdf.

Hyland, P., Shevlin, M., Fyvie, C., Cloitre, M., and Karatzias, T. (2019). The relationship between ICD-11 PTSD, complex PTSD and dissociative experiences. *Journal of Trauma & Dissociation*, 21 (1) 62–72.

Jovanović A. A., Dunjić B. D., and Milovanović S. D. (2016). Forensic Aspects of Post-Traumatic Stress Disorder in Martin, C. R., Preedy, V. R., & Patel, V. B. (Eds.). *Comprehensive guide to post-traumatic stress disorders*. Springer International Publishing. p: 77-96.

Kessler R. C., Sonnega A., Bromet E. Posttraumatic stress disorder in the National Comorbidity Survey. *Archives of General Psychiatry* 52:1048–60, 1995.

Kilpatrick, D. G., Resnick, H. S., Milanak, M. E., Miller, M. W., Keyes, K. M., & Friedman, M. J. (2013). National estimates of exposure to traumatic events and PTSD prevalence using DSM-IV and DSM-5 criteria. *Journal of Traumatic Stress*, 26(5), 537–547.

Kinzie, J. D., Boehnlein, J. K., Riley, C., & Sparr, L. (2002). The effects of September 11 on traumatized refugees: Reactivation of posttraumatic stress disorder. *Journal of Nervous and Mental Disease*, 190(7), 437441.

Lanska D. J. (2018). The Dancing Manias: Psychogenic Illness as a Social Phenomenon. *Frontiers of Neurology and Neuroscience*, 42:132-141.

Matto, M., McNiel, D. E., & Binder, R. L. (2019). *A Systematic Approach to the Detection of False PTSD.*

Mauritz, M. W., Goossens, P. J., Draijer, N., and Van Achterberg, T. (2013). Prevalence of interpersonal trauma exposure and trauma-related disorders in severe mental illness. European *Journal of Psychotraumatology*, 4(1), 19985.

Miller, H. A. (2005). The Miller-Forensic Assessment of Symptoms Test (M-FAST) test generalizability and utility across race literacy, and clinical opinion. *Criminal Justice and Behavior*, 32(6), 591-611.

Morgan, C. A., Feuerstein, S., Fortunati, F., Coric, V., Temporini, H., and Southwick, S. (2005). Posttraumatic stress disorder within the forensic arena. *Psychiatry* (Edgmont), 2(10), 21.

Paris, J. (2019). Dissociative identity disorder: validity and use in the criminal justice system. *BJPsych Advances*, 25(5), 287-293.

Pitman, R. K., Sparr, L. F., Saunders, L. S., and McFarlane, A. C. (1996). *Legal issues in posttraumatic stress disorder.*

Rocchio, L. M. (2020). Ethical and Professional Considerations in the Forensic Assessment of Complex Trauma and Dissociation. *Psychological Injury and Law*, 13: 124-134.

Rogers R., Sewell K. W., Goldstein A.: Explanatory models of malingering: a prototypical analysis. *Law & Human Behavior*, 18:543–52, 1994.

Şener, M. T., Şahingöz, S., Yücel, A., & Güleç, M. (2014). Fiziksel travmalara bağlı gelişen psikopatalojiler ve ve adli değerlendirmede önemi. *Adli Tıp Dergisi,* 28 (2): 108-114.

Sequeira A. J., Fara M. G., Lewis A. Ethical Challenges in Acute Evaluation of Suspected Psychogenic Stroke Mimics. *Journal of Clinical Ethics*, 2018 Fall; 29(3):185-190.

Smith, G. P., and Burger, G. K. (2003). Structured inventory of malingered symptomatology. *Journal of the American Academy of Psychiatry and the Law.*

Sparr, L., & Pankratz, L. D. (1983). Factitious posttraumatic stress disorder. *The American Journal of Psychiatry.*

Tjeltveit, A., and Gottlieb, M. (2010). Avoiding the road to ethical disaster: Overcoming vulnerabilities and developing resilience. *Psychotherapy Theory, Research, Practice, Training*, 47, 98-110.

Yadav, P. K. (2017). Ethical issues across different fields of forensic science. *Egyptian Journal of Forensic Sciences*, 7(1), 10.

In: Forensic Psychiatry …
Editor: Nursen Turan Yurtsever
ISBN: 978-1-53619-530-9

Chapter 6

SUBSTANCE USE DISORDERS

Necati Serkut Bulut* and Yıldız Akvardar
Department of Psychiatry, Marmara University,
School of Medicine, Istanbul, Turkey

ABSTRACT

In a time when addiction has become a global and growing public health problem with detrimental impacts on societies worlwide, it is more than necessary for contemporary health professionals to familiarize themselves with the basic concepts of substance use disorders. One substantial reason is that addiction and psychoactive substance use-related issues present in a wide range of medico-legal contexts within clinical settings. Among the most common examples of forensic practices are evaluations for addictions allegedly caused by inappropriate prescriptions; physicians' impairments due to substance abuse; civil law issues such as termination of the rights of addicted parents; and criminal law issues, including probation, coerced treatment, and evaluations for criminal responsibility. Aside from the theoretical struggles that result from the multifaceted nature of addictive phenomena, clinicians are also likely to confront numerous ethical dilemmas during their clinical assessment and decision-making process. These may include but are not limited to

* Corresponding Author's E-mail: serkutbulut@gmail.com.

conflicts regarding confidentiality, legal responsibilities, the obligation to act in the best interests of the patient, and informed consent procedures. Taken together, clinicians need to have a basic knowledge of addiction medicine, which is imperative to deal with the most common forensic challenges in the daily practice, and maintain their adherence to ethical standards.

INTRODUCTION

With the rapidly increasing prevalence of addiction and the multifaceted impacts on communities all over the world, the understanding of the basic concepts of addiction is becoming more than useful medical knowledge or a practical skill for health professionals. One substantial reason is that psychoactive substance use-related issues present in a wide range of medico-legal contexts, which might not exempt the physicianfrom liability in daily practice. Among the most striking examples of the forensic practices are assessments for addictions allegedly caused by inappropriate prescriptions; physicians' impairments due to substance abuse; civil law issues such as termination of the rights of addicted parents; and criminal law issues including probation, coerced treatment, and evaluations for criminal responsibility.

In this chapter, following a brief introduction of some of the basic concepts of substance use disorder, we aimed to provide a framework on the intersection between addiction medicine and forensic psychiatry, with an emphasis on related ethical challenges that clinicians may face during their daily practice.

DEFINITIONS AND CONCEPTUALIZATION OF ADDICTION

The American Society of Addiction Medicine defines addiction as "a treatable, chronic medical disease involving complex interactions among brain circuits, genetics, the environment, and an individual's life experiences." The definition also emphasizes that "people with addiction use substances or engage in behaviors that become compulsive and often continue despite harmful consequences" (Cunningham et al. 2020).

The reader should be aware that a multitude of complex models (and definitions) have been proposed for addiction, which in turn, yield great conceptual controversies even among major authorities and international health organizations. For instance, while the American Medical Association (AMA) defines dependence/addiction as a disease, theAmerican Psychiatric Association (APA) and the World Health Organization describe substance dependence as a mental disorder. From the biomedical perspective, addiction is seen as a "brain disease" like Alzheimer's dementia, and the emphasis is largely put on the neurobiological or physiological components, implying that addictive behavior is mostly automatic and beyond control or even inaccessible to "willpower." The psychological models, on the other hand, highlight that psychoactive agents are commonly used by vulnerable (e.g., certain personality types or those with specific personality traits or other psychopathology-generated emotional states) individuals as self-medication to deal with a deeper psychological problem, or they underscore the role of environmental factors (family, friends, overall permissiveness of cultures, policy measures, advertising, social media, etc.) in the development of addiction, as in the example of social learning theories (Adan et al. 2017; Carvalho et al. 2019).

Although both the brain and psychosocial factors are substantial components in the etiology of substance use disorders, conceptualizing addiction merely as a "brain disease" or a "psychological disturbance" is an overly reductionistic approach that overlooks the multifaceted and extremely complex nature of the phenomenon. From this viewpoint, the biopsychosocial model of substance use disorders, which is also largely in line with the traditional psychiatric paradigm, can provide a more comprehensive theoretical framework for addictive phenomena (Milhorn 2018).

TERMINOLOGY AND DIAGNOSTIC CLASSIFICATION

A perplexing nomenclature is used to describe the wide range of substance use-related problems such as substance/alcohol misuse, problematic use, risky use, abuse, dependence, addiction, etc. Moreover, this ambiguity does not seem to be limited to the lay use of these terms but is evident at even the highest scientific/academic levels (Kelly 2004).

When a physician is assigned as an expert for a forensic assessment by the court, he or she is thus required to be highly prudent regarding nuances and what is meant by the corresponding terminology (Beckson et al. 2003). The need for the use of a common language and standard criteria must be taken into consideration. The Diagnostic and Statistical Manual of Mental Disorders (DSM), the most popular diagnosis system for mental disorders, and the International Classification of Diseases (ICD) serve as the primary sources of reference within the framework of medico-legal practices for most cases. Hence, it is in the clinicians' best interests to familiarize him or herself with "DSM nomenclature" as well as the major changes that have appeared in the latest version of the manual (DSM-5, American Psychiatric Association, 2013). However, the conceptual discrepancies between the actual and the previous (DSM-IV) editions are beyond the scope of this chapter (Sokolov 2017). The keypoint for the reader is that the former DSM-IV diagnoses of "substance abuse" and "substance dependence" have been eliminated in DSM-5 and collapsed into a single "substanceuse disorder" diagnosis and are identified by eleven criteria (see Table 1). The diagnosis is now also accompanied by a severity specifier: a substance use is considered to be of mild severity when characterized by the presence of two to three symptoms, moderate by four to five, and severe by six or more symptoms out of eleven.

In sum, it is without a doubt that the use of standard criteria within the common framework of a diagnostic classification system (such as DSM or ICD) provides a myriad of advantages in medico-legal practices. However, regardless of the terminological modifications and conceptual shifts between different editions of these manuals, the take-home message for the reader is that the expert will be required to collect additional information from different modalities to build a decent clinical formulation because the information contained in a clinical diagnosis is barely satisfactory to address the questions of ultimate concern to the law (Miller 2010).

Table 1. Comparison of DSM-IV and DSM 5

DSM-IV		**DSM-5**	
Any 1 = Abuse	+	1. Failure to fulfill responsibilities	2 or more= Substance Use Disorder
	+	2. Use in physically hazardous situations	
	Legal Problems	3. Craving	Mild: 2-3 symptoms
	+	4. Social/interpersonal problems	
Any 3 = Dependence	+	5. Larger amounts or over longer period than intended	
	+	6. Unsuccessful efforts to cut down or control	Moderate: 4-5 symptoms
	+	7. A great deal of time spent	
	+	8. Giving up important activities	
	+	9. Ongoing use despite persistent problems	Severe: 6 or more symptoms
	+	10. Tolerance	
	+	11. Withdrawal	

+, criterion on the right applies to both.

ABOUT PSYCHOACTIVE SUBSTANCES

A psychoactive substance is defined as "a pharmacologically active, consumable material, usually self-administered, that can reliably have, among other physiological effects, a discernible impact on one's mood, emotions, feelings, sensations, perceptions, and/or thinking" (Aggarwalet al. 2012). Not surprisingly, the lack of theoretical consistency is also evident concerning the classification systems of psychoactive substances. In broad terms, the most common categories for psychoactive substances include (1) central nervous system (CNS) depressants such as alcohol, opioids, benzodiazepines, and barbiturates; (2) CNS stimulants such as cocaine, amphetamine and derivatives, nicotine, and caffeine; and (3) hallucinogens such as lysergic acid diethylamide (LSD), phencyclidine (PCP), and psilocybin. Cannabinoids, inhalants, and many other "designer" drugs (such as synthetic cathinones, phenethylamines, etc.) fall outside such a classification (Liechti 2015). Notably, only nine of these substance are enlisted in the DSM-5 (alcohol; caffeine; cannabis; hallucinogens; inhalants; opioids; sedatives, hypnotics, and anxiolytics; stimulants; and tobacco), and all are presented in separate sections (Grant and Chamberlain 2016).

Psychoactive substances are most commonly self-administered by inhalation, sniffing, ingestion, or intravenous injection. Their chronic use may result in impaired body functions, tissue damage, and/or characteristic bodily signs that, in some cases, are easily discernible by inspection, as in the example of needle marks in heroin use or "meth mouth" in methamphetamine addiction.

Knowledge of the pharmacokinetic and pharmacodynamic characteristics of a particular drug is essential in understanding the basics of the short- and long-term psychoactive effects associated with its use. The physician should consider that the intoxication symptoms for a certain substance administered at the same dose may vary greatly among users due to a multitude of individual differences (physiological and psychological) as well as environmental and other contextual (user's motivation, expectation, etc.) factors. The recognition of the wide range of potential psychoactive effects that an intoxicated individual may experience might therefore be of utmost concern for the expert during a forensic assessment. For instance, alcohol may interfere with the formation of episodic memory as in the case of alcoholic blackouts (Ewing et al. 2014). The use of cannabinoids can induce acute psychosis that may last beyond the period of intoxication or may later facilitate the development of a psychotic disorder (Wilkinson et al.2014). LSD is known to induce profoundly altered states of consciousness and is associated with vivid auditory and visual hallucinations (Mülleret al. 2017). Although transient in a large proportion, the use of methamphetamine may often cause acute symptoms of agitation, violence, delusions, etc. (Glasner-Edwards and Mooney 2014).

Assessment for Addiction and Treatment

When performing a forensic evaluation regarding substance use disorders, it is of paramount importance for the expert to gather information from all available medical records and collateral sources. APA's Practice Guideline for Treatment of Patients with Substance Use Disorders introduces an overview for the evaluation of a substance use disorder and suggests the following: "A systematic assessment of the mode of onset, quantity, frequency, and duration of substance use; the escalation of use over time; the motivation for use; the specific circumstances of the individual's substance use; the desired effect of the substance used; the most recent dose of each substance used; the time elapsed since the most recent use; the degree of associated intoxication; the severity of withdrawal syndromes; and the subjective effects of all substances used" (Kleber and McIntyre 2006; Kleber et al. 2007).

At the beginning of the evaluation for treatment, the clinician should first aim to build a trusting relationship and adopt a supportive, empathic, and nonjudgmental approach toward the patient. It should also be ensured that confidentiality, privacy, and dignity are respected in the setting where interviews take place (NICE pathways, 2018) (Nolanet al. 2018). During the evaluation, the APA Practice Guidelines suggest that the evaluator focus on the following areas: "a history of any prior treatment; modalities used, duration and dose of the treatment; level of adherence to the treatment; treatment outcomes from short to long-term as measured by subsequent substance use; level of general functioning achieved, etc. For individuals with a previous history of treatment, additional history may include the duration of abstinence, the factors that promoted abstinence, the factors associated with relapse, the individual's attitude toward prior treatment, and expectations about future treatments" (Kleber and McIntyre 2006; Kleber et al. 2007).

Laboratory Testing

The expert who assesses current or recent substance use in a suspected individual is required to be familiar with the basics of laboratory tests that are used in detecting psychoactive substance metabolites and associated biochemical alterations. Multiple alternative sources exist for biologic specimens, including urine, blood, saliva, hair, breath, sweat, and meconium. These various tissues and bodily fluids exhibit different rates and durations of excretion that result in different detection windows for substances. Blood has the the earliest and shortest windows of detection for substances (most are cleared at measurable levels in twelve hours or less). Urine's detection window is about one to three days for most substances, while cannabinoids may be detected in the urine for prolonged periods due to their fat solubility (up to one week for intermittent users, up to one month for daily users). A standard one-and-a-half-inch hair sample gives information over past three-month drug use (Hadland and Levy 2016).

Case 1

An inmate was brought to the hospital from the correctional facility with the institution's demand for medical assessment for suspected psychoactive use after four weeks following his incarceration. A urine test yielded a positive result for cannabinoids, although the patient claimed that he had last "smoked pot" a couple of days before his admission to the facility. A detailed interview revealed a history of frequent and long-term use of cannabis. The attendant officers also reassured the doctors that the correctional facility was highly secured, making access to any substance literally impossible, and reported in favor of a forced abstinence. Considering the patient's chronic pattern of use and the pharmacokinetic characteristics of cannabinoids (highly lipophilic profile leading to its storage in adipose tissue), the expert's opinion was that the positivity was most likely due to the delayed excretion of this particular substance. Indeed, the control test performed in the subsequent week turned out to be negative.

Forensic Implications of the Blood Alcohol Level

In the forensic evaluation of "driving under the influence" (DUI) cases and alcohol-related traffic injuries, it is of utmost importance to properly determine and interpret blood alcohol levels at the moment of the incident in order to assess criminal liability. From a forensic standpoint, the extent of the intoxication is primarily determined by the measurement of blood alcohol concentration (BAC) (Spitz 2010), a parameter that consists of various metrics, which may lead to confusion. The percentage or gram percent alcohol measurement actually indicates grams per 100 mL of a body fluid, usually the blood (i.e., the BAC). Thus, a BAC of 0.08%, the most common BAC indicator for DUI, is equivalent to 0.08 g%, 0.08 g/100 mL, 0.08 g/dL, 80 mg%, or 80 mg/dL of ethanol. Another measure is Promille, which is mostly popular in some European countries, with 1 Promille being equal to 1 gram of alcohol per 1 L of blood. That is to say, a BAC of 0.08% is equivalent to 0.8 Promille (Perry et al. 2017).

A "standard" drink contains around 14 g of pure ethanol. Examples of a standard drink are 330–350 mL (12 oz) of regular beer (usually 5% alcohol), 140–150 mL (5 oz) of wine (typically 12% alcohol), and 40–45 mL (1.5 oz) of distilled spirits (around 40% alcohol). Generally, it is estimated that one standard drink will produce a BAC of 0.02% (0.2 Promille) for a 90-kg (around 200-lb) male and 0.04% for a 56-kg (around 125-lb) female, whereas two and three drinks would result in a doubled and tripled BAC, respectively. The average blood ethanol disappearance rate (BEDR) is 121 mg/L per hour. BEDR ranges from 0.010 to 0.022% per hour for 95% of the population (Spitz 2010; Perry et al. 2017).

In moderate amounts, alcohol is mostly associated with euphoria and mild physiological changes such as dehydration and vasodilation, which result in bloodshot eyes and flushed skin. Clinical signs of moderate impairment may include relaxed demeanor, slowed movement, poor coordination, exaggerated gestures, etc. More severe intoxication symptoms usually occur at BAC levels higher than 0.08% and include incoherent and slurred speech, loss of balance, significantly impaired motor coordination, stumbling, agressive-hostile behavior, emotional lability, and disorientation. At higher concentrations (BAC higher than 0.4%), alcohol depresses the central nervous system, which may lead to coma and death due to central respiratory arrest.

Table 2. BAC Limits in Countries

Country	Illegal BAC limit
Argentina	0% for public transport and commercial vehicles, 0.02% for motorcycles, and 0.05% for all others
Australia	0% for provisional and professional drivers, 0.05% for all others
Canada	0.08%
China	0%
England	0.08%
France	0.02% for new drivers, 0.05% for others
Germany	0% for beginners or professional drivers, 0.03% if involved in a traffic offense or accident, 0.05% otherwise
India	0.03%
Iran	Not applicable (alcohol is banned)
Japan	0.03%
South Africa	0.02% for professional drivers, 0.05% for others
Spain	0.03% for new or professional drivers, 0.05% for others
Turkey	0% for commercial transport and public service drivers, 0.05% for others
USA	0.08% (depends on state)

Source: World Health Organization, Global Information System on Alcohol and Health, Alcohol Control Policies. Retrieved from https://apps.who.int/gho/data/view.main.54600.

The laws concerning DUI vary greatly between countries. Moreover, several types of legislation have been enacted to help control impaired driving. These include the BAC level established as illegal, the sanctions imposed for impaired driving under different circumstances, the use of rehabilitation programs for offenders, and the system for regranting the licenses of offenders whose driving privileges have been suspended or revoked (Stewart 2000). Major differences also exist concerning the fines and licensing sanctions that are established for impaired driving offenses

(Table 2). Depending on the BAC levels and whether or not the offender has had previous offenses, duration of the license suspension may range from months to several years; prison sentences are also possible in most countries.

In sum, one should consider that predetermined BAC limits do not legitimize driving under the influence of alcohol consumed in lesser amounts given the substantial individual differences that exist in the severity of impairment caused by alcohol. Moreover, research findings point out that impairment in handling emergency situations in traffic is evident for anybody and at almost any level.

TREATMENT MODALITIES IN ADDICTION AND COERCED TREATMENT

Although associated with high relapse rates, treatment for substance use disorders is effective, and the outcomes are comparable to those in other chronic medical diseases (McLellan et al. 2000). Considering the highly heterogeneous clinical presentation of the patients and the complex etiology of the phenomenon, a multimodal (i.e., biopsychosocial) approach remains the keystone of treatment for substance use disorders in most cases. The basic therapeutic steps involve performing an elaborate assessment, managing intoxication and withdrawal symptoms, addressing psychiatric and medical comorbidities, and implementing a well-defined treatment plan (Kleber and McIntyre 2006). Among the most common treatment settings are hospitals, residential facilities, partial hospitalization/day hospital treatment programs, outpatient programs, and correctional facilities for inmates. Psychosocial treatment approaches include individual and group therapies as well as self-help fellowships such as Alcoholics Anonymous. Medical/pharmacological treatments are often a major component of the treatment and are widely used to manage withdrawal syndromes, treat psychiatric comorbidities, or support abstinence, as in the case of methadone or buprenorphine for opiate use disorders or naltrexone, acamprosate, or disulfiram for alcohol use disorders (Kleber et al. 2007; Witkiewitz et al. 2019).

Unlike many other fields of medicine, treatment for substance use disorders may be legally mandated under a variety of circumstances, such as drug-related nonviolent offenses. In contrast with the traditional viewpoint, research findings indicate that the compulsory treatment does work and is as effective as treatment obtained voluntarily by highly motivated individuals (Miller and Flaherty 2000). In a typical setting, the patient must comply with the requirements of the treatment procedure and remain sober during the process in order to be exempted from criminal sentencing. These requirements generally involve periodic monitoring of the individual concerning his or her therapeutic motivation and regular participation in treatment per the physician's report as well as submission to regular mandatory urine tests for toxicological screening (Rosner 2003).

SUBSTANCE USE AND INFORMED CONSENT TO TREATMENT

In broad terms, the concept of informed consent requires that the consent be given voluntarily (voluntariness), the patient is sufficiently informed on the proposed treatment (disclosure), and he or she has the capacity to understand the provided information and make medical decisions (competence). Although the ethical underpinnings of the concept bring numerous theoretical and practical dilemmas that extend beyond the scope of this chapter, from the perspective of substance use disorders, the most recognized exceptions to informed consent are (1) incompetence: given that the patients are required to be "competent" in order to give informed consent, patients with substance use disorders have an increased risk of not being able to provide it at a certain moment due to the temporary impairment in their decisional capacity, as in the example of intoxication syndromes or psychotic states associated with drug use. In this case, substitute consent may be obtained from the next of kin or the court. (2) emergency medical situations: if an incapacitated patient presents with a medical emergency or imminent danger of serious harm to him or herself or to others due to acknowledged effects of a substance, the physician has the right to implement the appropriate treatment that is limited to the acute management of the condition, as in the case of delirium tremens or intoxication syndromes with violent behaviors and psychotic symptomatology, etc. Nevertheless, the definition of medical emergencies is far less clear in substance use disorders than in other fields of medicine. (3) coerced treatment: as the most common example of treatments without informed consent, in coerced treatments, the individual's autonomy (refusal of the treatment) is overridden by the judicial verdict (Loue 2010; Kambam 2017). Crucially, even if the individual is hospitalized by the court order within the context of coerced treatment, no treatment can be administered against a patient's will unless he or she is significantly incapacitated due to a psychotic state, delirium, intoxication, etc. (Evren and Öncü 2018).

CONFIDENTIALITY IN SUBSTANCE USE DISORDERS

The principle of confidentiality is crucial for building a therapeutic relationship between the physician and the patient with a substance use disorder. Maintaining confidentiality provides a solid base for the patient's autonomy, given that it is the patient him or herself who has the control of any information regarding his or her medical status or treatment. In the United Statesand many other countries, sensitive information, including the identity, diagnosis, and treatment episodes of those who have alcohol and drug problems, is protected by licensing and confidentiality laws. While divulging such information is largely precluded, there are acknowledged circumstances that exist where disclosing confidential patient information to a third party is associated with "overriding public interest," as in the example with licensing authorities. Among other exceptions that take priority over the privacy/confidentiality principle within the context of substance use treatment are disclosure enforced by court orders or statutory provisions; disclosure to seek consent from the next of kin to provide medical intervention; and disclosure in the presence of any other overriding legal, moral, or social necessities, such as reporting child abuse, crime against treatment personnel, murder, etc. (Beran 2010; Miller2010; Sadoff 2011).

SUBSTANCE USE AS A RISK FACTOR FOR CRIME

There is ample evidence that substance use is associated with an increased tendency for violence for any individual, with the risk being even more significant for those with a psychiatric comorbidity. In jail populations, it has been reported that the inmates with a history of alcohol abuse were more likely to have committed a violent offense. Moreover, around three-fourths of all inmates with a history of drug abuse reported having used a substance in the month prior to arrest (Belenko 2000). Considering this close relationship between addiction and violence, it is also imperative for the expert to assess a patient's future dangerousness during his or her forensic evaluation and provide appropriate treatment alternatives. In cases where the risk for violence seems to be imminent, it is again the clinician's duty to "take reasonable steps" toprotect a potential victim from a patient who presents a significant threat (Miller 2010). On the other hand, clinicians are also *bound* by the ethical and legal licensure to uphold *confidentiality. They are* legally restrained from disclosing information that was shared within the protected client-counselor relationship, implying that the attempt to prevent violence may result in a violation of confidentiality (Vanderpool 2011). In sum, there remains substantial ethical and legal controversies for physicians regarding in what situations a duty exists, what is predictable, and what is meant by "reasonable steps" (Beckson et al. 2003).

Case 2

A 35-year-old male was brought to emergency room by the police after exhibiting physically violent behaviors in a pub. His sister stated that before leaving the house the patient had consumed a liter of vodka earlier that evening. They learned that he had a long ongoing history of alchohol abuse, which became dramatically severe over the last two years, with recurrent outbursts of anger and alcoholic blackouts. At the time of admittance to the hospital, the patient seemed to be confused, had difficulties standing upright, and exhibited slurred speech. His blood ethanol concentration was 220 mg/dL. As the emergency doctor took him to a separate room for physical examination, the patient suddenly began to cry and stated that he had recently hit and killed someone with his car when he was drunk. He admitted that he could no longer bear the burden of this guilt but that he didn't want anyone else to know about it.

SUBSTANCE USE AND CRIMINAL RESPONSIBILITY

In American and European common law, voluntary intoxication does not provide an alibi for an individual who has committed a crime, although it is possible for the involuntary intoxication to be considered "legally excusable" in some particular circumstances. The latter crucially requires that the offender has consumed the substance in question due to enforcement or trickery or exhibited violent behaviors due to a previously unknown susceptibility to an atypical but recognized effect of the substance or an idisosyncratic intoxication caused by a drug prescribed as a treatment. If the long-term substance use has resulted in irreversible and permanent brain damage that presents with psychiatric symptoms or cognitive deficits, it is possible in some jurisdictions to come up with an "insanity defense" within the context of "settled insanity." However, temporary psychotic states caused by voluntary administration of a substance fall outside this framework (Slovenko 1995; Beckson et al. 2003).

The assessment for the criminal responsibility of an individual with a history of substance use necessitates knowledge of the effect of the particular substance on this individual's mental functions at the time of the alleged crime. On the other hand, considering that the effects elicited by psychoactive substances may vary greatly between individuals, the expert should build his or her diagnostic approach on findings and facts that are as objective as possible. The assessment should therefore address but not remain limited to (1) whether the individual's psychotic symptoms were only present during the intoxication or they persisted for periods extending beyond the pharmakokinetic characteristics of the drug or (2) evidence indicating that the psychotic symptoms were present before or at times other than the intoxication period (Feix and Wolber 2007).

Landmark Case (Montana v. Egelhoff)

In July 1992, James Egelhoff (defendant) was convicted of deliberate homicide after police found him drunk in a car next to his gun with two victims who both had been shot to death. Egelhoff claimed that his state of intoxication made him incapable of committing such a crime and that he was not able to remember what happened that night. Although the Montana Supreme Court later reversed the guilty finding, the U.S. Supreme Court subsequently reversed the appeal on certiorari and convicted Egelhoff of murder. The Court's decision was based on common law arguments to hold that the exclusion of evidence on "voluntary intoxication" was not a violation of due process (Ford and Rotter 2014).

Addiction as an Outcome of Medical Treatment

In some cases, litigations against health professionals may include allegations that (1) a physician's prescriptions have caused a patient's addiction, (2) the patient was not adequately informed of the risks of the medication, (3) substance use comorbidity was not adequately assessed, or (4) the substance use disorder was not appropriately treated. Inappropriate prescription of controlled pharmaceuticals (prescribing excessive amounts of medications or prescription of such agents to a patient with known substance use disorder) puts the physicians at risk of losing their prescribing rights as well as their professional license (Rosner 2003).

Case 3

A 38-year-old male patient with a past history of multiple substance use and antisocial personality disorder (with several criminal records) sued all ten physicians working in the emergency department of a state hospital on the grounds that they had caused him to become “an opiate addict.” The examination of the patient’s medical records by the assigned expert revealed that he had been admitted to the emergency department due to his reported symptoms of renal colic on an almost daily basis for the past two months. The expert also noticed that the staff had often mentioned the patient’s threatening and demanding behaviors for the intramuscular administration of pethidine on the grounds that his pain would not resolve otherwise. Due to the physicians’ working shifts, the patient had met with more than ten physicians, against whom he later filed an action for damage alleging malpractice and demanded financial compensation.

Case 4

A 35-year-old male general surgeon was noticed behaving overly strange for several weeks. His colleagues and the surgery team members reported that he mostly seemed indifferent to his surroundings and was less talkative than ever. He was often late to work for no apparent reason, left the operating room several times, and was absent for hours in some cases. He had problems sustaining his attention and made a critical mistake that almost caused a fatal injury during his last surgery. In the same period, a routine check of the medication inventory revealed a significant shortage in the number of alfentanil ampoules, a short-acting synthetic opioid analgesic. The nurse in charge remembered unexpectedly seeing the doctor leave the medical supply room in a hurry just a few days before the incident.

Not surprisingly, physicians are mostly unwilling to report colleagues’ substance use for understandable reasons. However, the AMA’s Principles of Medical Ethics (American Medical Association 2001) states that “it is unethical for a physician to practice medicine while under the influence of a substance which impairs the ability to practice." Furthermore, it is an ethical obligation for medical doctors to report impaired colleagues according to the AMA Principles of Medical Ethics (American Medical Association 2001; Beckson et al. 2003; Miller 2010). That is, if a physician has concerns about a colleague's functional impairment due to a substance use disorder, he or she has the responsibility to intervene as quickly as possible. In the United States, Physicians Health Programs (PHPs) serves as a confidential resource for healthcare professionals suffering from substance use disorders and other potentially impairing conditions. In such a situation, it is best for a physician to contact a PHP to report a colleague with a suspected substance abuse. While the United States and a few other countries have addressed the problem since the '70s, most European countries still have no national or hospital policy to deal with impaired physicians. According to European directives on workers' health and safety, the occupational health physician entrusted with the medical surveillance of hospital workers is often mandated to manage impaired professionals (Magnavita 2006).

CONCLUSION

In summary, there are a variety of instances in which health workers become involved in ethical conundrums where substance abuse issues present within the medico-legal context. Clinicians need to have the basic skills, competency, and professional knowledge that are imperative to deal with the most common examples of forensic challenges in the daily practice. In doing so, one should also strive to maintain his or her objectivity, honesty, and neutrality during evaluations as well as to adhere to the ethical principles.

REFERENCES

Adan, A., Forero, D. A. and Navarro, J. F. (2017). Personality traits related to binge drinking: a systematic review. *Frontiers in psychiatry,* 8, 134.

Aggarwal, S. K., Carter, G. T., Zumbrunnen, C., Morrill, R., Sullivan, M. and Mayer, J. D. (2012). Psychoactive substances and the political ecology of mental distress. *Harm Reduction Journal,* 9, 4.

Akvardar, Y., Türkcan, A. and Cakmak, D. (2002). Is substance abuse among physicians a problem? *Turkish Journal of Psychiatry,* 13, 238-244.

Beckson, M., Bartzokis, G. and Weinstock, R. (2003). Substance abuse and addiction. In *Principles and Practice of Forensic Psychiatry, 2Ed*, pp. 694-706, CRC Press.

Belenko, S. R. (2000). *Drugs and drug policy in America: A documentary history*. Greenwood Press Westport, CT.

Beran, R. G. (2010). Privacy within the First Decade of the Twenty-First Century. In *Principles of Addictions and the Law*, pp. 75-80. Elsevier.

Carvalho, A. F., Heilig, M., Perez, A., Probst, C. and Rehm, J. (2019). Alcohol use disorders. *The Lancet,* 394, 781-792.

Cunningham, C., Edlund, F. M. J., Fishman, M., Gordon, D. A. J., Jones, D. H. E., Langleben, D., Meyer, M., Springer, S., Woody, F. G. and Femino, J. *The ASAM National Practice Guideline for the Treatment of Opioid Use Disorder: 2020 Focused Update.*

Evren, C. and Öncü, F. (2018). Forensic Psychiatry Practices in Alcohol and Substance Use and Addiction (Alkol-Madde Kullanımı ve Bağımlılığı ile ilgili Adli Psikiyatri Uygulamaları). *Practice Guideline For Forensic Psychiatry (Adli Psikiyatri Uygulama Kılavuzu), 3Ed,* 145-95, Ankara: Türkiye Psikiyatri Derneği Yayınları.

Ewing, S. W. F., Sakhardande, A. and Blakemore, S. J. (2014). The effect of alcohol consumption on the adolescent brain: A systematic review of MRI and fMRI studies of alcohol-using youth. *NeuroImage: Clinical,* 5, 420-437.

Feix, J. and Wolber, G. (2007). Intoxication and settled insanity: a finding of not guilty by reason of insanity. *Journal of the American Academy of Psychiatry and the Law Online,* 35, 172-182.

Ford, E. B. and Rotter, M. (2014). *Landmark Cases in Forensic Psychiatry.* New York: Oxford University Press, USA.

Glasner-Edwards, S. and Mooney, L. J. (2014). Methamphetamine psychosis: epidemiology and management. *CNS drugs,* 28, 1115-1126.

Grant, J. E. and Chamberlain, S. R. (2016). Expanding the definition of addiction: DSM-5 vs. ICD-11. *CNS spectrums,* 21, 300-303.

Hadland, S. E. and Levy, S. (2016). Objective testing: urine and other drug tests. *Child and Adolescent Psychiatric Clinics,* 25, 549-565.

Kambam, P. (2017). Informed consent and competence. In *Principles and practice of forensic psychiatry, 3Ed,* pp. 115-124, CRC press.

Kelly, J. F. (2004). Toward an addictionary: A proposal for more precise terminology. *Alcoholism Treatment Quarterly,* 22, 79-87.

Kleber, H. D. and McIntyre, J. S. (2006). *Practice Guideline for Treatment of Patients with Substance Use Disorders.* American Psychiatric Association Arlington, VA.

Kleber, H. D., Weiss, R. D., Anton, R. F., George, T. P., Greenfield, S. F., Kosten, T. R., O'Brien, C. P., Rounsaville, B. J., Strain, E. C. and Ziedonis, D. M. (2007). Treatment of patients with substance use disorders, American Psychiatric Association. *The American journal of psychiatry,* 164, 5-123.

Liechti, M. E. (2015). Novel psychoactive substances (designer drugs): overview and pharmacology of modulators of monoamine signalling. *Swiss medical weekly,* 145, w14043.

Loue, S. (2010). Bioethical Decisions, Substance Use and Addiction: The Clinical Context. *Principles of Addictions and the Law*, pp. 81-96.

Magnavita, N. (2006). Management of impaired physicians in Europe. *La Medicina del lavoro,* 97, 762.

McLellan, A. T., Lewis, D. C., O'brien, C. P. and Kleber, H. D. (2000). Drug dependence, a chronic medical illness: implications for treatment, insurance, and outcomes evaluation. *Jama,* 284, 1689-1695.

Milhorn, H. T. (2018). Definitions of Substance Dependence. *Substance Use Disorders*, pp. 17-24.

Miller, N. S. (2010). *Principles of addictions and the law: applications in forensic, mental health, and medical practice*. Academic Press.

Miller, N. S. and Flaherty, J. A. (2000). Effectiveness of coerced addiction treatment (alternative consequences): A review of the clinical research. *Journal of substance abuse treatment,* 18, 9-16.

Müller, F., Lenz, C., Dolder, P., Lang, U., Schmidt, A., Liechti, M. and Borgwardt, S. (2017). Increased thalamic resting-state connectivity as a core driver of LSD-induced hallucinations. *Acta Psychiatrica Scandinavica,* 136, 648-657.

Nolan, K., Shearn, P., Gholitabar, M. and Richardson, J. (2018). *NICE public health guidance update.* Oxford University Press.

Perry, P. J., Doroudgar, S. and Van Dyke, P. (2017). Ethanol forensic toxicology. *Journal of the American Academy of Psychiatry and the Law,* 45(4), 429-438.

Rosner, R. (2003). *Principles and practice of forensic psychiatry, 2Ed,* CRC Press.

Sadoff, R. L. (2011). Ethical Issues in Forensic Psychiatry in the United States. *Ethical Issues in Forensic Psychiatry: Minimizing Harm*, 3-26.

Slovenko, R. (1995). *Psychiatry and criminal culpability*, John Wiley and Sons.

Sokolov, G. (2017). Substance abuse and addiction. In *Principles and Practice of Forensic Psychiatry, 3Ed,* pp. 815-822, CRC Press.

Spitz, W. U. (2010). Forensic Considerations in Blood Alcohol Evaluation. In *Principles of Addictions and the Law*, pp. 167-175. Elsevier.

Stewart, K. (2000). *On DWI laws in other countries.* DIANE Publishing.

Vanderpool, D. L. (2011). 13 Risks of Harm to the Forensic Expert: the Legal Perspective. *Ethical Issues in Forensic Psychiatry*, 197-211, John Wiley and Sons.

Wilkinson, S. T., Radhakrishnan, R. and D'Souza, D. C. (2014). Impact of cannabis use on the development of psychotic disorders. *Current addiction reports,* 1, 115-128.

Witkiewitz, K., Litten, R. and Leggio, L. (2019). Advances in the science and treatment of alcohol use disorder. *Science Advances,* 5(9), eaax4043.

In: Forensic Psychiatry …
Editor: Nursen Turan Yurtsever
ISBN: 978-1-53619-530-9

Chapter 7

EVALUATION OF INTELLECTUAL DISABILITIES

Onur Tugce Poyraz Findik and Ayşe Burcu Erdoğdu*

Department of Child and Adolescent Psychiatry,
School of Medicine, Marmara University,
Pendik Research and Training Hospital, Istanbul, Turkey

ABSTRACT

Individuals who have limited communication skills, poor memory, and decreased social reasoning skills are those who have intellectual disability (ID) and have special needs in the criminal justice system as well as in many aspects of their lives. The disability in intellectual skills includes a wide range in the developmental spectrum from mild to severe and requires comprehensive evaluations for each category. Individuals with ID are more often victims of crime compared to individuals without ID. However, they also have increased vulnerability in committing crimes. In terms of social rights, many countries have treatment services and legal regulations for individuals with ID. Although the legal regulations for ID individuals are quite old historically, there continues to be difficulties in identifying individuals with ID and the need to improve the understanding

* Corresponding Author's E-mail: onurtuuce@hotmail.com.

of their needs in different stages of the justice system. This chapter contains information about the definition of ID, its scope, the diagnostic process, how individuals with ID are involved in criminal justice, and recommendations on how to conduct a forensic interview that addresses the developmental, social, and emotional needs of individuals with ID. It also focuses on the differential diagnosis of malingering and ID with the use of clinical evaluations and test batteries.

Introduction

Although the prevalence of intellectual disability (ID) in the population varies across countries, it is estimated to be around 1 percent (Zablotsky et al. 2019; McGuire et al. 2019; Maulik et al. 2017). Individuals with ID are often found in the justice system as victims of crime; however, studies report that the prevalence of ID in the criminal justice setting varies between 2 and 10 percent (Lindsay 2011). Many countries have treatment services and legal regulations for individuals with ID. If it is suspected that a defendant is suffering from mental health problems, a mental health examination can be requested. However, the lack of understanding of mental illness and difficulties in the evaluation process pose a serious challenge to the criminal justice system (Seay 2006).

The presentation of ID varies widely. ID individuals are generally considered to have a disorder that makes their functionality, behavior control, and understanding of social situations and laws difficult for them (Marti-Agusti et al. 2019). They may not be able to understand abstract concepts and complex information. Because their knowledge and judgment about moral concepts and social situations may be limited, they may have difficulty making judgments about right and wrong. This does not mean that they cannot distinguish between right and wrong but that they have difficulty adapting and applying these concepts to new situations in their lives. Because of the desire to be socially accepted by others and to please others, they are open to changing their mind without correctly evaluating social situations. Their limited communication skills, impaired reasoning skills, dependency on others to survive, and ability to be manipulated can contribute to their committing criminal acts (Seay 2006; APA 2013). In addition, individuals with ID are more likely to suffer from comorbid psychiatric disorders than the general population (APA 2013; Dekker and Koot 2003). Mental health problems such as substance abuse and psychotic disorders are more prevalent in individuals with ID than those without (Plant et al. 2011; Morgan et al. 2008). The presence of comorbid psychiatric disorders makes impulse control more difficult. On the other hand, when individuals with ID commit a crime, their vulnerabilities have an impact on the court's evaluation process. They can be exempted from punishment or practices such as a reduction in their penalties can be made on the grounds that they have no criminal responsibilities. However, when an individual with ID commits a criminal activity, the extent to which ID contributes to the crime by disrupting the ability to comprehend the nature and consequences of the crime and to establish causality must be determined (Davis and Lister 2019).

It is suggested that individuals with ID have no higher crime rates than the general population. However, some authors state that their crime characteristics are different. The antisocial behaviors associated with violent crimes, sexual crimes, fires, and substance addiction are especially emphasized. When the relationship between intelligence quotient (IQ) and crime is examined, it is estimated that committing a crime is exceedingly rare in those with an IQ less than 50. On the other hand, those with borderline IQ were found to have more frequent sexual crime and burglary than the general population, but more serious crimes such as murder or armed robbery were less in this group. Moreover, criminal justice and other practices for ID are considered to have a great impact on the prevalence of crime among individuals with ID and the types of crimes they commit (Simpson and Hogg 2001).

Another important emphasis in this area is that individuals with ID should not be directly exempted from prosecution. There may also be individuals with ID who can understand the consequences of crime and carry out legal processes. The cases where individuals try to imitate ID to reduce the severity of punishment is a serious challenge for law enforcement and mental health professionals (Seay 2006). During the judging process, it is important to determine how the event in question was affected by the presence and severity of ID. Each individual should be evaluated separately, and which aspects of the individual's ID affect which aspects of the individual's behavior should be dealt with separately (Davis and Lister 2019).

The Definition and Diagnosis of ID

The condition called ID is what was formerly known as mental retardation. Although the name has changed with the publication of the Diagnostic and Statistical Manual of Mental Disorders, Fifth Edition (DSM-5), the scope is the same. In this text, the terms ID and mental retardation are used synonymously. Three basic criteria are evaluated for the diagnosis of ID. These are limited intellectual functions, impaired adaptative functioning, and the early onset of symptoms (APA 2013).

Intellectual functions are also called intelligence, and this term includes mental skills such as learning, reasoning, planning, problem-solving, abstract thinking, understanding complex ideas, etc. (APA 2013; Singh 2016). One method of measuring intellectual functions is IQ tests. In order to measure IQ correctly, a psychometrically valid, culturally appropriate, and individually applied tool is required. IQ test results are represented along the (bell-shaped) curve where the normal mean value is 100. Individuals with ID have usually placed two standard deviations below the mean (IQ below 70) (APA 2013). Various problems (i.e., speech problems, sensory or motor difficulties) can affect the assessment, and the individualized test is chosen taking these into account. A frequently used IQ test for children in our country is the Wechsler Intelligence Scale for Children-Revised form (WISC-R) (Kaufman 1975). It provides verbal IQ, performance IQ, and total IQ scores. Nowadays, WISC-IV and the new version WISC-V have started to be applied. The adult version is available for people over sixteen years old. Based on the current population, IQ tests are periodically reshaped in line with cultural changes and needs.

Adaptive functioning is based on the sum of conceptual (language and literacy; money, time, and number concepts; mathematics; memory; knowledge, etc.), social (empathy, interpersonal skills, ability to make and maintain friendships, social judgment, obeying rules/laws, and avoiding victimization), and practical skills (self-management skills such as personal care, health care, travel, professional skills, routines, telephone use, money management) that are learned, applied, and developed in daily life (APA 2013). However, when evaluating ID, additional factors such as the age and cultural characteristics of the society in which the individual lives should also be taken into account. Criminal behavior and other problematic behaviors should not be considered an indicator of adaptive functioning difficulties. At this point, it is important to distinguish "adaptive" functioning difficulty or deficiency from "maladaptive" behavior (Ellis et al. 2017). It is important to collect information from third parties for the evaluation of adaptive functioning. For this purpose, the evaluation process is strengthened by using multiple sources of information and approaches, including the observation of the individual in various settings and activities (Seay 2006). In forensic evaluations, the relationship of informants with the individual and possible interests should be taken into account. Gathering information from multiple sources and applying different approaches can help to overcome this problem. Expertise-based knowledge and clinical experience of professionals working in this field gain importance. Also, it is beneficial to use records such as school records, hospital documents, social service information, and previous criminal records and previous forensic psychiatric interviews, if any, that support the persistence of symptoms since early developmental stages (Seay 2006). Additionally, it should not be forgotten that besides their limitations in their skills, individuals may have strengths in some areas. As a result, a versatile assessment is required to determine whether an individual has ID.

With the publication of DSM-5, the most striking change in addition to the name change of mental retardation was the abandonment of IQ scores as diagnostic criteria. This encouraged the view of a more comprehensive evaluation of the individual's ordinary life skills. The terms mild, moderate, severe, and profound are used to describe the symptom severity. Grouping is done by focusing on daily life skills rather than a specific IQ score (APA 2013).

Mild Intellectual Disability

Most people (about 85 percent) with ID are classified as mildly intellectually disabled. It is usually noticed in the period of the beginning of school. Speech delay may occur. Individuals with mild ID have difficulty learning concepts that cover one or more of the concepts such as reading, writing, arithmetic, time, or money. Also, they may have difficulty with communication skills. They use more immature and concrete language than their peers and cannot show expected age-level skills in understanding and reasoning social situations. These individuals can learn practical life skills that allow them to function in life with minimal support (APA 2013). Generally, their IQ tests are often in the 50–69 range. They may have literacy skills at the primary school level, and they can later get a job by gaining skills with special education.

Moderate Intellectual Disability

Individuals with moderate ID may have limitations in understanding, language skills, self-care, and motor skills. Over time, they can learn the necessary self-care, social adaptation, and communication skills that are needed for daily life. They constitute about 10 percent of all individuals with ID. Their self-care requires moderate support (APA 2013), and they often have IQ scores in the 36–49 range. They can gain academic skills at the first grade level of primary school, but their educational goals are generally aimed at gaining daily life skills. They can eventually work with support and in simple jobs.

SEVERE INTELLECTUAL DISABILITY

Severe ID presents with serious developmental delays. Children in this group are usually diagnosed very early. They have obvious motor retardation. They can usually understand what is spoken, but other than that, they have limited communication skills. They may gain late speaking skills or may not gain any at all. They need supervision in social settings and often need institutional care or family care to live. They cannot learn to read and write (APA 2013).

Although the definition and scope of ID are clear in mental health discipline, there are important difficulties about how to evaluate it in the justice system. As well as the victimization of these individuals, the risk factors that cause them to be involved in crime and the difficulties encountered in the evaluation process are prominent issues.

LEGAL REGULATIONS REGARDING ID IN THE HISTORICAL PROCESS

Historically, crimes have been evaluated in terms of their consequences, regardless of whether there is a relationship between the condition of the person and the crime. In this case, whether it is an animal, a child, or a mentally ill person that committed the crime, the perpetrator has been held responsible for the crime. The first practices regarding the relationship between crime and imperfection took place in Roman law. Roman criminal law chose to subject the mentally ill person to similar provisions as minors in terms of punishment. In the historical process, there are also special regulations in Islamic law regarding situations such as mental illness that affect the will of the individual (Ünver Y 1989). Similarly, today we see that legal liability related to ID is handled with special regulations in many countries. Situations such as criminal liability, legal responsibilities such as marriage and divorce, and the perception of the moral evil of an event require different evaluations in individuals with ID.

Children with ID and Forensic Interviews in the Juvenile Justice System

Case 1

A fourteen-year-old girl, Ayse, was referred to our child and adolescent psychiatry clinic to assess the reliability/credibility of her account that she had been sexually abused by her step-grandfather. The incident was reported to the police when Ayse told her teachers at the school that her "grandfather is a pervert" and that he touched her chest and between her legs. In the evaluation of the child's mental state, it was observed that she had age-appropriate physical development, her self-care was moderate, her verbal communication skills were limited, and she was willing to cooperate with the interviewer. The child made statements about the incident such as "my grandfather touched me," "he's always doing it," "he kissed my lips once," "we were in the bedroom," "he made me touch men's dick," and "he was sticking his dick to my butt." It was observed that she had difficulty remembering details such as the time and place of the event. Her father said that Ayse had been quiet recently, looked unhappy, and did not want to go to her grandfather's house. Ayse had never told her father about the incidents until that day because she was afraid of his possible reactions. It was thought that Ayse had moderate ID due to her difficulty in remembering the details about the event, limited verbal skills, and use of a simpler and concrete language for her chronological age. Her IQ test score was also appropriate for a moderate ID diagnosis. Although there were occasional inconsistencies in her statements about the incident, it was thought that the child was subjected to sexual abuse due to the fact that the sexual knowledge she had was incompatible with her age and developmental level. A report was drawn up stating that the child's statement on this matter could be credited.

Case 2

A seventeen-year-old boy, Ahmet, was referred to court after he tried to forcefully kiss his girlfriend in class and touched her private parts. A forensic assessment was requested on whether Ahmet perceived the legal meaning and consequences of the sexual assault crime. It was learned that Ahmet had a genetic diagnosis of deletion in the long arm of chromosome 4 and could not speak until the age of three and a half. In addition, his walking was delayed and he had been in special education since the preschool period and learned to read and write late. The current academic skill of the child was at the third grade primary school level. He was having problems making money calculations and could do simple addition and subtraction with finger calculations. Ahmet had been having difficulty controlling his sexual impulses since he entered adolescence and had been using psychotherapy and medication for a long time to manage his impulse control, which included outbursts of anger. During the interview, Ahmet gave short answers to the questions asked about the incident, missed eye contact, and said that he regretted it. He was able to give partially correct answers to the questions that evaluated his social reasoning skills. Ahmet's IQ test and examination findings made us think that he had mild ID. A report was prepared that Ahmet, who had difficulty in impulse control, did not develop the ability to manage his behavior and did not perceive the legal meaning and consequences of his behavior.

Case 3

Sevgi, a fourteen-year-old girl, was referred to our clinic by the court to assess whether a guardian should be appointed to her. Sevgi, who had been under the care of social services for about a year and was receiving special education, was evaluated together with the caretaker at her institution. Sevgi was taken under institutional care while living with her family because her mother had left home and her father had difficulty providing care. During her stay in the institution, Sevgi was able to dress herself, eat her own food, stand alone in the room, and go out to the garden alone, but she had difficulties in fine motor skills such as tying shoelaces. In addition, she could not do toileting and bathing alone, and she could not go to the market alone or calculate money. However, Sevgi was in harmony with her friends in the institution, she was participating in activities during the day, and she could initiate mutual social communication herself. She was cooperative and smiled during the mental evaluation. She gave simple answers to questions and knew the days and months with help, but her concept of what year it was was not yet developed. She could not remember the names of the people who were with her but continued to talk using words such as "doctor" and "manager." The child's thought content was limited, but she had partial insight. She could not recognize letters and numbers, count to ten, write her name, or do simple addition. She could not adapt to the applied IQ tests. Based on the information given by the institutional staff and clinical observation, she was thought to have moderate ID. A report was prepared stating that Sevgi had moderate ID; therefore, she was limited in exercising her civil rights and in constant need of help. Since she did not endanger the safety of others, there was no benefit in a court hearing.

Individuals with ID have cognitive delays, reasoning difficulties, and limited communication skills. They are likely to be exposed to bullying, violence, discrimination, and maltreatment throughout their lives (Newlin et al. 2015). Often they cannot get enough education and leave school early. Some may have been trained in institutional care, and some may have limited verbal capacity. As a result, they may not have access to information that other individuals can understand and may not know how to defend themselves through legal means. In the justice system, they may encounter professionals who do not have knowledge and experience about the behavior and needs of ID individuals and may have difficulties accessing justice for all these reasons (Mental Disability Advocacy Center 2017). These make ID individuals vulnerable as crime victims. Studies have shown that children with disabilities are three to four times more likely to be a victim than their nondisabled peers (Sullivan and Knutson 2000; Jones et al. 2012).

Individuals with ID deal with the justice system in various ways, not only as victims but in many other situations. They may be a witness, defendant, convicted criminal, or eyewitness or have interests in the proceedings or be alleged guilty. A mental health professional may be asked for an opinion on whether an ID criminal has sufficient comprehension skills for judgment, whether his or her statements are invalid due to the limitations arising from ID, or whether he or she has sufficient understanding of the legal rights of the person. Whatever the purpose of the assessment, the role of the judicial interview is to use scientific data, experience, and expertise to assist the court in making a decision in a case (Salekin et al. 2010).

The legal system recognizes that a defendant must be shown to have committed a crime (actus reus) and must intend to take such an action (mens rea) to be held criminally responsible for the crime. Criminal responsibility assessments are conducted to help the judge to what extent mental health symptoms affect the mood of the accused at the time of the crime and the relationship between this effect and criminal responsibility. In these evaluations, it is primarily investigated whether the reported symptoms meet the definition of mental illness. Then, justified determinations are presented about the effect of this situation on the person's skills, behavior, and judgment processes at the time of the crime (Davis and Lister 2019).

Criminal responsibility assessments are one of the most controversial judicial evaluations. Criminal responsibility can be defined as the responsibility to act in accordance with the law. For a person who does not act in accordance with the law to be punished, it is expected that he or she has reached a certain level in terms of age and mental-intellectual-physical maturity; knows the meaning of his or her action, its consequences, and the meaning of these according to the social value judgments; and had free will when he or she performed the action (Ünver 1989). Children can acquire the skills required for criminal responsibility as a result of brain maturation that occurs with age, and after acquiring these skills, they can be held responsible for their actions. According to the Turkish Penal Code, children cannot be punished for any crime before they turn eleven. However, after they turn twelve, they can be considered criminally responsible for their actions. The evaluation process of criminal responsibility is comprised of the child's mental and physical development, the age at the time the crime was committed, whether he or she has a mental disorder, whether he or she knows the nature of the act and whether it is a crime, whether the child has reached the mental development milestone to know that others will be harmed and he or she will be punished as a result of the action, the way the crime was committed, the emotional conditions, and the sociocultural framework. In this context, it is expected that the criminal responsibility of individuals with ID will be affected at different rates. This evaluation process requires the knowledge and experience of professionals from special expertise such as forensic medicine, neurology, or child and adolescent psychiatry.

Criminal responsibility assessments are often a multistep process to present an objective assessment that comprehensively addresses available clinical data and legal problems. These evaluations focus on whether the defendant can be held criminally responsible for his or her actions at the time of the crime. Determining the diagnosis related to the mental health problems is necessary; however, it is not the last step. Once the diagnosis is clear, it should be examined whether it has an impact on the crime in question and whether this effect is at a level that should be taken into account (Ferguson and Ogloff 2011). These assessments are retrospective and are often performed months after the crime. For this reason, offenders can forget important details from that period. In this respect, past records can be useful in helping them remember (such as what was said to the police at the time of the arrest). The past records should be carefully evaluated, but it should be considered that there is the possibility that they may not be able to fully describe their mental state, there may be a lack of knowledge (such as being under the influence of a substance), and they might not be able to fully express their symptoms (Davis and Lister 2019). Interviews with additional sources such as family members may be required for diagnosis and background information. These additional sources may be inclined to exaggerate the defendant's symptoms to obtain facilities associated with a disability determination. Evaluators should evaluate the data they obtain and keep these possibilities in mind. It is also useful to evaluate the motivational sources that pushed the person to commit the crime. Criminal liability should be investigated separately for each type of crime. Malingering is more common than treatment-oriented interviews to gain an advantage in criminal liability assessments. This is an important aspect of forensic evaluation that is different from diagnostic and therapeutic evaluation (Davis and Lister 2019).

It is also important to know how to obtain correct information from individuals with ID in a forensic interview. Forensic interviews can often shed light on different aspects of the trial process and reveal new aspects of the committed crime (Newlin et al. 2015). Forensic interviews with children with ID may require some special concerns. A forensic interview with a child is a process where developmental and evidence-based methods are applied by experienced people to obtain legally meaningful information. A report should be prepared after the tests required for forensic assessment, investigation of past records, and interviews are completed. Professionals working in this field should generally be upto date on services available for people with mental disabilities and the laws governing these services and be able to provide advice when necessary.

Some important issues to be considered during the forensic interview with children with ID are as follows:

1. The interview should be held in a child-friendly, safe, and comfortable environment.
2. As should be done for every child, the interviewer should perform developmental screening for the child with a developmental disability (Anderson 2006).
3. Forensic interviews with children with developmental delays require different knowledge and experience than those with typically developing children. It may be helpful to collect some important information before the interview. The interviewer should have information about the child's disability. Arrangements appropriate to the child's disability may be necessary for the interview environment. For example, for a child with limited speaking skills, it may be necessary to have some nonverbal auxiliary tools such as dolls and drawing materials in the interview environment. Especially in situations related to sexual abuse, dolls

and drawings can be useful in re-enacting the event or determining the details (Ballard and Austin 1999).

4. ID does not mean that a person looks younger than someonehis or her own age. The skills of people with disabilities may differ during different times of their life. They may have acquired some skills with time, training, and experience (Anderson 2006). This should be taken into account in the forensic evaluation process.
5. Some children may need more time to feel comfortable during the interview. It can be started by talking about everyday events that will not bother the child. For example, it might help to talk about theirpets, hobbies, sports, etc. At this stage, the interviewer gets the opportunity to evaluate the child's developmental level, understanding capacity, and language use (Ballard and Austin 1999). Inappropriate questions about developmental characteristics will result in missing information.
6. The cultural background of the child has an impact on the child's language use, behavior toward foreigners, and perception of his or her experiences (Newlin et al. 2015; Ballard and Austin 1999). An interview that is not sensitive to cultural characteristics can lead to misunderstandings.
7. In conditions where judicial capacity is being assessed, the child's level of knowledge of basic concepts such as legal terms and court proceedings should be assessed. He or she may be asked to answer some specific questions about legal issues related to the alleged crime.
8. The interviewer should make sure that he or she understands the child well and that the child understands the details of the interview correctly. For this purpose, short questions such as "You said... .Did I get that right?" and "Did it make sense to you this way?" may be asked (Anderson 2006).
9. Each child has different and unique characteristics. Different children who have experienced the same life events will reveal different symptoms with the effect of different genetic, cultural, and temperament-associated factors (Newlin et al. 2015).

10. It is helpful to find out what the child thinks about lying and its consequences. At this stage, it might be a good idea to introduce and give examples about the concepts of true and false and to ask the child questions regarding these concepts. For example, interviewers might ask "It's rainy today. Do you think this is true or false?" The child can also be asked what he or she thinks about the consequences of lying. After talking about the concepts of truth and lying, the child's understanding might be strengthened by asking "Shall we make an agreement that we will only talk the truth here?" (Ballard and Austin 1999).
11. Repetitive questions and repeated interviews with multiple interviewers can be harmful. Children with disabilities change their answers more when asked repetitive questions compared to their peers (Henry and Gudjonsson 2003). This results in inconsistency in expressions. Children with ID may be slow to process information, recall it from memory, and form responses. For this reason, it may be necessary to wait a few seconds after asking a question. It may also take time for some children to cooperate and become comfortable with the interview. In such cases, multiple non duplicative interviews can be performed (Anderson 2006; Newlin et al. 2015).
12. Questions in forensic interviews should be open-ended. Obtaining the child's free-recall memory-based information is the most important milestone in the forensic interview. Open-ended questions should be used for this purpose, and the children should be encouraged to answer questions such as "Can you tell me all that happened?" and "Can you tell me more about that?" in as much detail as possible. In this part, there should not be any input that interrupts the child's orientation or speech. More focused questions may be asked in the later stages of the interview (Newlin et al. 2015). However, cognitive slowness and memory deficits of children with ID may play a critical role in the recall phase. In addition, in those who can remember accurately and in detail, the

interviewer may encounter problems arising from communication problems.

13. While yes/no questions are less preferred in all forensic interviews, they may cause different difficulties in this group. In a study conducted with individuals with ID, it was found that people with a low IQ have a high tendency to answer "yes" (Sigelman et al. 1981). To overcome this difficulty, it may be helpful to give the instruction that it is appropriate for the child to answer "I don't know" during the interview when he is unsure (Anderson 2006).
14. Multiple-choice questions may be a better alternative to yes/no questions (Heal and Sigelman 1995). For example, the interviewer could ask "You said you were home when it happened. Who else was with you—your mother, father, brother, or anyone else?"
15. When asking questions, the developmental period and skills, not the chronological age, should be taken into consideration. The interviewer should consider limited cognitive skills, and the questions may need to be asked more concretely, more structured, and more clearly than usual. For example, he or she may need to ask "Where did he touch?" "What did he say to you?" or "What were you wearing?"
16. Hesitations and silences should be allowed, and in such cases, the child should not be asked to focus on the issue quickly (Newlin et al. 2015).
17. When ending the interview, the child should be asked whether he or she has anything else to say. When leaving, his or her effort must be appreciated.

Differential Diagnosis of Malingering and ID

Due to the criminal liability in courts and the earnings obtained by issuing medical reports in hospitals, it has become important to distinguish the individual with ID from malingered ID. This situation gains social importance when disability programs, insurance systems, and labor constraints are considered. In evaluations regarding ID, accompanying systems such as school records, academic skills, and peer relations should also be addressed in addition to the intellectual capacity and adaptive functioning of the individual. In the psychiatric examination, the development of test batteries that can be used in the clinic and the determination of cut-off scores have come to the forefront in order to make the differential diagnosis of malingering and ID (Rogers 1992;Hayes, Hale, and Gouiver 1998; Schretlen and Arkowitz 1990). In the studies conducted in this area, it has been shown that test batteries such as the Minnesota Multiphasic Personality Inventory, the Structured Interview of Reported Symptoms, and the Malingering Scale can be used to distinguish between malingering and ID. In addition, the malingered ID group has been found to show more personality pathology compared to ID individuals (Schlesinger 2003). A further step in the distinction between malingered ID and ID may be hospitalization and follow-up and rehabilitation (Anderson and Hewitt 2002).

CONCLUSION

Intellectual disability is identified by a weakness in intellectual functions and adaptation problems and is stratified in terms of severity. It is grouped by mild, moderate, and severe ID in which the prevalence in the population decreases and disability increases, respectively. While individuals with intellectual disability are less involved in serious crimes, it is important to determine the intelligence levels of these people in the prosecution and judgment process.

REFERENCES

American Psychiatric Association. (2013). *Diagnostic and statistical manual of mental disorders (DSM-5®).* Washington, DC: American Psychiatric Pub.

Anderson, J. (2006). *Forensic interviews of children who have developmental disabilities*. Update, *19*(1).

Ballard, M. B. & Austin, S. (1999). Forensic interviewing: Special considerations for children and adolescents with mental retardation and developmental disabilities. *Education and Training in Mental Retardation and Developmental Disabilities*, *34* (4), 521-25.

Davis, K. M. & Lister, M. B. (2019). Conducting Disability Evaluations with a Forensic Perspective: the Application of Criminal Responsibility Evaluation Guidelines. *Psychological Injury and Law*, *12*(1), 52-63.

Dekker, M. C. & Koot, H. M. (2003). DSM-IV disorders in children with borderline to moderate intellectual disability. I: Prevalence and impact. *Journal of the American Academy of Child & Adolescent Psychiatry*, *42*(8), 915-22.

Ellis, J. W., Everington, C. & Delpha, A. M. (2017). Evaluating Intellectual Disability: Clinical Assessments in Atkins Cases. *Hofstra L. Rev*, *46*, 1305.

Ferguson, M. & Ogloff, J. R. (2011). Criminal responsibility evaluations: Role of psychologists in assessment. *Psychiatry, Psychology and Law*, *18*(1), 79-94.

Hayes, J. S., Hale, D. B. & Gouvier, W. D. (1998). Malingering detection in a mentally retarded forensic population. *Applied Neuropsychology*, *5*(1), 33-6.

Heal, L. W. & Sigelman, C. K. (1995). Response biases in interviews of individuals with limited mental ability. *Journal of intellectual disability research*, *39*(4), 331-40.

Henry, L. A. & Gudjonsson, G. H. (2003). Eyewitness memory, suggestibility, and repeated recall sessions in children with mild and moderate intellectual disabilities. *Law and Human Behavior*, *27*(5), 481-505.

Jones, L., Bellis, M. A., Wood, S., Hughes, K., McCoy, E., Eckley, L. & Officer, A. (2012). Prevalence and risk of violence against children with disabilities: a systematic review and meta-analysis of observational studies. *The Lancet*, *380* (9845), 899-907.

Kaufman, A. S. (1975). Factor analysis of the WISC-R at 11 age levels between 61/2 and 161/2 years. *Journal of Consulting and Clinical Psychology*, *43*(2), 135.

Lindsay, W. R. (2011). People with intellectual disability who offend or are involved with the criminal justice system. *Current Opinion in Psychiatry*, *24*(5), 377-81.

Martí-Agustí, G., García-Largo, L. M., Martin-Fumadó, C., Martí-Amengual, G. & Gómez-Durán, E. L. (2019). Intellectual disability: Criminality, assessment and forensic issues. *Spanish Journal of Legal Medicine*, *45*(4), 155-62.

Maulik, P. K., Mascarenhas, M. N., Mathers, C. D., Dua, T. & Saxena, S. (2011). Prevalence of intellectual disability: a meta-analysis of population-based studies. *Research in developmental disabilities*, *32*(2), 419-36.

McGuire, D. O., Tian, L. H., Yeargin-Allsopp, M., Dowling, N. F. & Christensen, D. L. (2019). Prevalence of cerebral palsy, intellectual disability, hearing loss, and blindness, National Health Interview Survey, 2009–2016. *Disability and health journal*, *12*(3), 443-51.

Mental Disability Advocacy Center. (2017). *Access to Justice for Children with Mental Disabilities: International Standards and Findings from Ten EU Member States, 2015*. Retrived from: http://www.mdac.org/sites/mdac.info/files/access_to_justice_children_ws2_standards_and_findings_english. Pdf.

Morgan, V. A., Leonard, H., Bourke, J. & Jablensky, A. (2008). Intellectual disability co-occurring with schizophrenia and other psychiatric illness: population-based study. *The British Journal of Psychiatry*, *193*(5), 364-72.

Newlin, C., Steele, L. C., Chamberlin, A., Anderson, J., Kenniston, J., Russell, A. & Vaughan-Eden, V. (2015). *Child forensic interviewing: Best practices.* Washington, DC: U.S. Department of Justice, Office of Justice Programs, Office of Juvenile Justice and Delinquency Prevention, Juvenile Justice Bulletin (No. NCJ 248749). Retrieved from https://ojjdp.ojp.gov/sites/g/files/xyckuh176/files/pubs/ 248749.pdf.

Plant, A., McDermott, E., Chester, V. & Alexander, R. T. (2011). Substance misuse among offenders in a forensic intellectual disability service. *Journal of Learning Disabilities and Offending Behaviour*, *2* (3), 127-35.

Rogers, R., Bagby, R. M. & Dickens, S. E. (1992). *Structured interview of reported symptoms (SIRS) and professional manual*. Odessa, FL: Psychological Assessment Resources.

Salekin, K. L., Olley, J. G. & Hedge, K. A. (2010). Offenders with intellectual disability: Characteristics, prevalence, and issues in forensic assessment. *Journal of Mental Health Research in Intellectual Disabilities*, *3*(2), 97-116.

Schlesinger, L. B. (2003). A case study involving competency to stand trial: Incompetent defendant, incompetent examiner, or "malingered by proxy"? *Psychology, Public Policy, and Law*, *9*(3-4), 381-399

Schretlen, D. & Arkowitz, H. (1990). A psychological test battery to detect prison inmates who fake insanity or mental retardation. *Behavioral sciences & the law*, *8*(1), 75-84.

Seay, O. J. (2006). Evaluating mental retardation for forensic purposes. *Applied Psychology in Criminal Justice*, *2*(3), 52-81.

Sigelman, C. K., Budd, E. C., Spanhel, C. L. & Schoenrock, C. J. (1981). When in doubt, say yes: Acquiescence in interviews with mentally retarded persons. *Mental retardation*, *19*(2), 53.

Simpson, M. K. & Hogg, J. (2001). Patterns of offending among people with intellectual disability: A systematic review. Part I: Methodology and prevalence data. *Journal of Intellectual Disability Research*, *45*(5), 384-96.

Singh, N. N. (2016). *Handbook of evidence-based practices in intellectual and developmental disabilities*. Switzerland: Springer International Publishing.

Sullivan, P. M. & Knutson, J. F. (2000). Maltreatment and disabilities: A population-based epidemiological study. *Child abuse & neglect*, *24*(10), 1257-73.

Ünver, Y. (1989). *Mental Illness and Its Effect on Criminal Liability in Criminal Law (Ceza Hukukunda Akıl Hastalığı ve Ceza Sorumluluğuna Etkisi). Unpublished Master Thesis*. Istanbul: University Institute of Social Sciences.

Zablotsky, B., Black, L. I., Maenner, M. J., Schieve, L. A., Danielson, M. L., Bitsko, R. H., Blumberg, S. J., Kogan. M. D. & Boyle, C. A. (2019). Prevalence and trends of developmental disabilities among children in the United States: 2009–2017. *Pediatrics*, *144* (4), e20190811.

In: Forensic Psychiatry …
Editor: Nursen Turan Yurtsever
ISBN: 978-1-53619-530-9

Chapter 8

DEMENTIA DISORDERS

Hatice Omercikoglu Ozden* and Nese Tuncer
Department of Neurology, Faculty of Medicine,
University of Marmara, İstanbul, Turkey

ABSTRACT

Dementia is the acquired, widespread, and often progressive impairment of cognitive functions that affects content rather than consciousness. Although its frequency increases with age, dementia is not always a condition that accompanies aging. Dementia is a condition that affects the cerebral cortex, its subcortical connections, or both. Minor neurological function changes may occur in memory and other cognitive areas with normal aging. Differentiating between normal aging and dementia is important for the beginning of the treatment and the social life of the patients and their families. Dementia is divided into primary neurodegenerative dementia and secondary forms of dementia (non-neurodegenerative) according to the underlying etiology and mechanism of dysfunction. Dementia is a chronic disease that mostly affects the elderly population and requires long-term care. It is important to make a good differential diagnosis regarding the patient's symptoms and not to miss the treatable causes of dementia. For now, as there are no disease-modifying

* Corresponding Author's E-mail: hozden@marmara.edu.tr.

treatments available for degenerative dementias, it is important to recognize and treat neurological and neuropsychiatric symptoms and to improve the quality of life of both the patient and the caregiver. When evaluating a patient with a complaint of forgetfulness, a detailed mental examination, cognitive tests, imaging, and laboratory tests should be performed. To protect patients and their relatives, the diagnoses and decisions should be recorded with all examinations. This chapter presents a practical and informative approach to the evaluation of a patient with a dementia.

INTRODUCTION

The World Health Organization describes dementia as a syndrome in which there is deterioration in cognitive function beyond what might be expected from normal aging. Memory, thinking, orientation, comprehension, calculation, learning capacity, language, and judgment are affected, and there is impaired ability in performing daily activities. Consciousness is not affected. Cognitive impairment is often accompanied by impaired emotional control, social behavior, or motivation. The *Diagnostic and Statistical Manual of Mental Disorders, Fifth Edition* (*DSM-V*) was published by the American Psychiatric Association (APA) in 2013 and the name of the "delirium, dementia, amnestic and other cognitive disorders" category was changed to "neurocognitive disorders." Dementia was renamed "major neurocognitive disorder" in the *DSM-V*, which also recognizes earlier stages of cognitive decline as "mild neurocognitive disorder" (see Table 1).

Fifty million people have dementia, and there are nearly ten million new cases worldwide every year. Dementia prevalence has risen to 7 percent of individuals above the age of sixty-five, and in developed countries there is a slightly higher prevalence (8 to 10 percent) due to longer life spans (Gale 2018). The incidence is higher in women and increases with age.

Table 1. Neurocognitive Disorders as Diagnosed in *DSM-5*

Diagnostic Major Neurocognitive Disorder/Dementia Mild Neurocognitive Disorder/MCI Criteria	
A Significant cognitive decline in one or more cognitive domains, based on: 1. Concern about significant decline, expressed by individual or reliable informant or observed by clinician 2. Substantial impairment, documented by objective cognitive assessment	Modest cognitive decline in one or more cognitive domains, based on: 1. Concern about mild decline, expressed by individual or reliable informant or observed by clinician 2. Modest impairment, documented byobjective cognitive assessment
B Interference with independence in everyday activities	No interference with independence in everyday activities, although these activities may require more time and effort, accommodation, or compensatory strategies
C Not exclusively during delirium	
D Not better explained by another mental disorder	

(Adapted from American Psychiatric Association. *Diagnostic and Statistical Manual of Mental Disorders. 5th Edition.* Arlington (VA): American Psychiatric Association; 2013).

CLASSIFICATION OF DEMENTIA

Dementia is divided into two main groups according to the underlying etiology and mechanism of dysfunction (see Table 2).

1. Primary neurodegenerative dementia
2. Secondary forms of dementia (non-neurodegenerative)

Neurodegenerative dementia is selective neuronal death that occurs in sensitive regions that are functionally related. In dementia in which cognitive impairment is prominent among neurodegenerative dementias, there are also dementia-plus syndromes characterized by the presence of extrapyramidal, pyramidal, cerebellar, autonomic signs, or symptoms before dementia with dementia or in the early clinical course (Gale 2018).

Table 2. Classification of Dementia

Primary Neurodegenerative Dementia	Secondary Forms of Dementia (Non-Neurodegenerative)
1. Alzheimer's Disease	1. Vascular Dementia
2. Lewy Body Dementia	2. Normal Pressure Hydrocephalus
3. Frontotemporal Dementia	3. Metabolic Causes
	4. Depression and Bipolar Disorder
4. Multiple System Atrophy	5. Vitamin Deficiency (B12, Thiamine, Niacin, Folic Acid)
	6. Neoplastic/Traumatic Brain Injury
5. Huntington's Disease	7. Vasculitides (Primary Vasculitis of the Central Nervous System, SLE-Related, Behcet Disease)
	8. Autoimmune Causes
6. Parkinson's Disease Dementia	9. Infectious Causes
	10. Toxic Causes (Lead, Arsenic, Organophosphate Pesticides)

Common causes of secondary forms of dementia that may occur throughout life include vascular, normal pressure hydrocephalus, metabolic, autoimmune, neoplastic/traumatic, infectious, intracranial masses, traumatic brain injury, psychiatric illness, vasculitides, and toxic and vitamin deficiency (Gale 2018).

EVALUATION AND DIAGNOSIS OF DEMENTIA

A detailed clinical history, neurological and mental status examination, laboratory tests, and structural brain imaging should be performed for the evaluation and diagnosis of dementia patients.

The history is clinically important and should be obtained from both the patient and the patient's relative, friend, or caregiver. History should characterize what the core symptom is and how it progresses, the course of symptoms, and how much higher cortical functions affect daily living activities. Information about vascular risk factors, use of medications, and current brain disorders should be asked in the history. There are many conditions that mimic dementia that may be overlooked during evaluation and, if detected, are potentially reversible. Additionally, attention should be paid to hearing and vision problems that can contribute significantly to cognitive impairment (Arvanitakis 2019).

A mental status examination helps to determine whether the level of consciousness or content is impaired and whether the cognitive dysfunction is global or limited. Multiple domains of mental function, including basic attention, memory, visual-spatial abilities, and executive function, should be assessed in a mental status examination (Arvanitakis 2019).

The Mini-Mental State Examination is a frequently used screening test used to evaluate cognitive function in daily practice, but it varies according to education level and is less sensitive to the presence of mild cognitive impairment (MCI) (Salem 2015). The other commonly used test is the Montreal Cognitive Assessment, which is useful in the early detection of cognitive impairment, including MCI with executive dysfunction. Neuropsychological tests are useful when decisions are not made by clinical evaluation and screening tests (Nasreddine 2005).

A neurological examination should be performed to detect neurocognitive problems such as aphasia, apraxia, and agnosia and to look for neurological focal signs and parkinsonism (Arvanitakis 2019).

Table 3. Clinical Evaluations of Suspected Dementia

- Taking detailed history from both the patient and the family
- Physical examination, neurological examination, and mental state examination
- Neuropsychological testing
- Chronic diseases, medications, drug blood levels (if possible), and family history
- Laboratory tests: hemogram, sedimentation, blood glucose level, electrolytes, kidney function tests, vitamin B12, folic acid, thyroid function tests, serological tests (HIV, VDRL, etc.)
- Structural brain imaging with CT or MRI
- If needed: EEG, LP, functional imaging

Laboratory tests required for the differential diagnosis of dementia include a hemogram, sedimentation, glucose, electrolytes, kidney function tests, vitamin B12, folic acid, thyroid function tests, serological tests, etc.

Computed tomography (CT) or magnetic resonance imaging (MRI) should be done for structural brain imaging. If specific etiology is suspected, electroencephalography (EEG), lumbar puncture (LP), and functional neuroimaging tests such as positron emission tomography (PET) should be performed (Arvanitakis 2019). The clinical evaluations and examinations that should be done in the patient with dementia are given in Table 3.

NEURODEGENERATIVE DEMENTIAS

Alzheimer's Disease

Alzheimer's disease (AD) is a neurodegenerative process, the cause and pathogenesis of which are not fully explained, and it is the most common cause of dementia. AD has a prevalence of 5 to 6 percent in individuals aged sixty-five and over, and its prevalence doubles every five years over the age of sixty-five (Gale 2018).

AD is usually sporadic; however, in 5 percent of cases, a genetic basis can be diagnosed, and the disease is genetically heterogeneous. Autosomal dominant inherited genes protein (APP), presenilin 1, and presenilin 2. The presenilin 1 gene mutation is associated with early onset (35–55 years old) AD. Genetic factors can also determine susceptibility to AD without direct cause. In late-onset AD, the risk of being affected and age of onset are linked to the number of apolipoprotein that have been shown to be associated with AD include amyloid precursor E (APOE) alleles on chromosome 19. In the APOE gene, three variables, e2, e3, and e4, are the single greatest risk for sporadic AD compared to non-e4 carriers (Scheltens 2016).

The main feature of AD pathology is the accumulation of abnormally folded Aβ and tau proteins in amyloid plaques and neuronal tangles. Aβ peptide originates from the APP, a transmembrane protein found in many tissues. Amyloid peptides (Aβ40 and Aβ42) and the abnormal accumulation of forty or forty-two amino acids form amyloid plaques. In AD, amyloid is deposited around the meningial and cerebral vessels and in gray matter. Neurofibrillary tangles, which are composed of paired helical filaments consisting of hyperphosphorylated tau, are fibrillar introcytoplasmic structures inside neurons. Although neurofibrillary tangles are not specific for AD, they first appear in the hippocampal formation; neurofibrillary tangles can then be seen in the entire cerebral cortex (Scheltens 2016).

CLINICAL SIGNS AND SYMPTOMS

Although the primary complaint of the patients with AD is not memory impairment, most patients have memory impairment at presentation. Episodic memory is mostly affected in patients with AD and semantic memory is affected in the later stages of the disease. Episodic memory is also divided into instant recall and recall of near events and more distant events. Short-term memory loss is associated with the hippocampus, entorhinal cortex, and medial temporal lobe, and it deteriorates significantly in the early period of AD. Instant memory is mostly associated with the prefrontal cortex and can be preserved for a long time (Peters 2009).

Executive function disorders in the early stages of AD can range from mild to more severe dysfunction. A decrease in the patient's insight and disorders in abstract thinking ability begin to appear. As the disease progresses, the inability to complete tasks occurs. Anosognosia, "lack of insight," is a common but variable feature in AD in which the patient can ignore their problems. Therefore, history should be taken from a relative who knows the patient. Over time, the loss of insight progresses and may cause behavioral changes after a while. Those with preserved insight are more prone to depression, and those whose insight is impaired may exhibit agitation, disinhibition, and psychotic symptoms (Barrett 2005).

In the middle and advanced stages of AD, neuropsychiatric symptoms are common. The first symptoms are apathy, social withdrawal, and irritability. While evaluating behavioral disorders such as agitation, aggression, and psychosis, the doctor should evaluate the patient in detail and consider the accompanying medical illness, drug toxicity, and other causes of delirium (Barrett 2005).

Apraxia is defined as an impairment in the functioning of learned motor tasks and disorder in the ability of practicing movements. Apraxia occurs after memory and language dysfunction in the later stages of AD. An apraxia examination involves asking the patient to pretend to use the tools she or he uses daily (Parakh 2004).

Changes in sleep patterns, early awakenings, and a decrease in total sleep time are common findings in AD. These findings occur in very early stages of the disease when there is no cognitive impairment yet (Yo-el S 2014).

In the early stages of AD, the neurological examination is normal. If pyramidal and extrapyramidal findings, myoclonus, and seizures are detected in the early period, other causes should be investigated in the etiology. Primitive reflexes and incontinence are mostly seen in advanced stages of AD (McKhann 1984).

Atypical Forms of Alzheimer's Disease

Classical progressive amnestic dementia findings are not found in a minority of patients. It can be difficult to determine whether these patients suffer from other types of dementia. Neuropathological examinations performed in these patients can reveal Alzheimer's pathology with atypical neuroanatomical distribution (Ridgway 2012).

Primer Progressive Aphasia

Primer progressive aphasia is characterized by progressive impairment of language functions in the early stage of the disease in which memory and other cognitive functions are preserved. There are three types of aphasia: non-fluent, semantic, and logopenic. Aphasia is associated with frontal lobe dementia rather than AD pathology; however, AD pathology was detected in a third of the patients in autopsy results. The type likely to be seen in AD is the logopenic variant in which the patient has difficulty finding words and understanding grammatical errors (Mesulam 2008).

Posterior Cortical Atrophy

Visual disorders such as visual-spatial perception disorder, simultanagnosia, contractional apraxia, oculomotor apraxia, optic ataxia, alexia, right-left disorientation, acalculia, limb apraxia, agraphia, and finger agnosia are observed in posterior cortical atrophy. However, anterograde memory function, speech-language functions, executive functions, behavior, and personality should be relatively preserved (Crutch 2017).

Frontal Variant of Alzheimer's Disease

AD has significant deficits in executive functions and behavioral problems compared to amnesia in the frontal variant. It may be difficult to differentiate frontal variant AD and behavioral variant frontotemporal dementia (FTD), especially in the early stages of the disease, according to their clinical presentation.

It is not uncommon for AD to coexist with other types of dementia. Vascular dementia is the most common type of dementia expected to occur with AD.

Lewy Body Dementia

Lewy Body Dementia (LBD) is the second most common cause of neurodegenerative dementia after AD (McKeith 2004). The main component of Lewy bodies is a protein called alpha-synuclein, which is known to play a role in axonal transmission. The abnormal alpha-synuclein protein accumulates in the cytoplasm, causing neurotoxicity and cell death. Spongiform vacuolization; loss of neurons in cholinergic, dopaminergic, noradrenergic, and serotonergic nuclei; and gliosis are also seen in neuropathology. Dopaminergic and cholinergic neurotransmitter losses are thought to be associated with Parkinsonism and cognitive disorders in LBD. Neuropathology is accompanied by findings in AD pathology in approximately 75 percent of cases. There are two different neuropathological subtypes with LB and amyloid plaques seen together (75 percent) and pure LB pathology (25 percent).

Clinical findings are evaluated in five groups: cognitive, neuropsychiatric, motor, sleep, and autonomic. According to the consensus criteria for the diagnosis of LBD, which were defined by McKeith et al. in 1996 and revised in 1999 and 2005, together with dementia, at least two of the major criteria, such spontaneous Parkinsonism, visual hallucinations, and fluctuation in course, make the diagnosis of "probable LBD."

LBD cognitive findings begin insidiously and progress slowly. Primary memory and language functions are relatively preserved. Parkinsonism seen in LBD usually has symmetrical and axial features. L-dopa response is usually not good in the early stages of the disease, or it begins to disappear shortly after the onset of the disease. LBD patients have severe neuroleptic sensitivity to conventional neuroleptics even at extremely low doses. This deterioration in Parkinsonism may be accompanied by impaired consciousness, autonomic findings, and neuroleptic malignant syndrome. Hallucinations, delusions, and depression are the most prominent neuropsychiatric features of LBD. Hallucinations are mostly stereotypic, detailed, well formed, and visual (Hanağası 2013). Fluctuation in cognition is the distinct change in alertness or cognitive and functional performance over a period of minutes, hours, days, or weeks. Fluctuation in clinical course is seen in 50 to 75 percent of patients (Hanson 2009). Sphincter defect, impotence, and orthostatic hypotension are autonomic findings seen in LBD. Autonomic findings are present from the onset of the disease and are more common than in PD. Rapid eye movement (REM) sleep behavior disorder is a common symptom in diseases with prominent "synucleopathy" pathology, such as LBD, PD, and multiple system atrophy. Insomnia, obstructive sleep apnea, central sleep apnea, and restless legs syndrome are other sleep disorders that can be seen in patients with LBD (Hanson 2009).

There are no specific bio-markers for LBD in serum, urine, and cerebrospinal fluids. Hippocampus and medial temporal lobe atrophy are less common in LBD than AD on cranial MRI. In the electroencephalography examination, slowing and temporary temporal slow wave activity can be seen from the early stage of the disease. Polysomnography is useful in showing REM sleep behavior disorder and other sleep-related clinical disorders that can be seen on the LCD. In brain metabolism studies, it has been shown that patients with LBD have significant parietal and occipital hypometabolism (Lobotesis 2001). In dopaminergic SPECT examination, there is caudate and putaminal hypometabolism in patients with LBD, and it is especially useful in differential diagnosis (Lobotesis 2001).

Frontotemporal Dementia

Frontotemporal dementia (FTD), one of the most common early-onset dementias, is a disease characterized by progressively worsening behavior and language disorders associated with degeneration in the frontal and anterior temporal lobes. More than 40 percent of patients diagnosed with FTD have a family history, and approximately 10 percent of these have an autosomal dominant inheritance. Familial transmission is most frequently observed in the behavioral variant FTD and FTD-ALS complex. Twelve genes currently associated with FTD have been identified; the two most common are microtubule-associated protein tau and progranulin (Miller 2019). Phenotypes of FTD such as age of onset, brain atrophy, clinical features, and disease duration may be affected by genetic factors.

The clinical presentation of FTD can be divided into two main groups—behavioral and language disorders. Language variants of FTD are divided into two groups such as nonfluent-agrammatic primary progressive aphasia (nfvPPA) and semantic primary progressive aphasia (Sivasathiaseelan 2019).

Behavioral Variant FTD

Behavioral disinhibition; apathy; loss of empathy; perseverative, stereotypic, or ritualistic behaviors; hyperorality; and changes in dietary habits are the main clinical features of patients in the early stages of behavioral variant FTD (bvFTD). The neuropsychological profile is an executive disorder in which visual-spatial functions and episodic memory are relatively preserved. Along with the neuropsychological profile, the presence of at least three of the six basic features is sufficient for a possible diagnosis of (bvFTD). There is a degree of frontal and/or temporal lobe atrophy, usually worse on the right, on a cranial MRI, and functional neuroimaging (FDG-PET or HMPAQ-SPECT) shows frontotemporal hypometabolism (Sivasathiaseelan 2019).

Nonfluent-Agrammatic Variant Primary Progressive Aphasia

Agrammatism and motor speech disorders are typical clinical features of nfvPPA. Agrammatism is a form of speech and often writing that typically consist of short, simple phrases that lack grammatical morphemes. Speech apraxia, which occurs as an articulation disorder, accompanies a slow speech that requires effort. Speaking speed is reduced, and prosody is impaired. Left fronto-insular atrophy is seen as a slight left sylvian fissure enlargement in axial sections in the early period on cranial magnetic resonance imaging (MRI). As the disease progresses, left frontal opercular and anterior insular atrophy becomes evident in the coronal sections (Sivasathiaseelan 2019).

Semantic Variant Primary Progressive Aphasia

Anomie and impairment in single word comprehension are the main features in semantic variant primary progressive aphasia. However, at least three diagnostic features such as loss of object information, preserved repetition, preserved motor speech and grammar, surface dyslexia, and dysgraphia must be present. Imaging-assisted diagnosis is made by demonstrating anterior temporal atrophy, hypometabolism, or hypoperfusion with at least one structural and/or functional imaging (Sivasathiaseelan 2019).

Multiple System Atrophy

Multiple system atrophy (MSA) is a sporadic and rapidly progressive neurodegenerative disease. There is abnormal deposition of the protein alpha-synuclei in the central and peripheral autonomic nervous system.

MSA is mainly characterized by various combinations of parkinsonism, cerebellar, pyramidal, or autonomic system symptoms and signs. There are two main clinical presentations: Parkinsonism findings are predominant in approximately 80 percent of patients, and cerebellar findings are predominant in 20 percent of patients (Wenning 2007). Although dementia is not one of the main features of MSA, patients may have varying degrees of cognitive deficits and personality and mood changes. Personality changes occur as apathy, passivity, emotional lability, and depression. Frontal-executive dysfunction is the most common presentation of cognitive disorder in MSA, and memory and visuospatial abilities may also be impaired. Therefore, all MSA patients should be evaluated for cognitive impairment (Brown 2010).

Parkinson's Disease Dementia

Even in the early stages of PD, varying degrees of cognitive impairment can be detected. Cholinergic, dopaminergic, and other monoaminergic systems are affected in patients with Parkinson's disease dementia (PD-D) (Emre 2007). In patients with PD-D, dopaminergic deficiency executive dysfunction; cholinergic deficiency, memory, attention, and executive dysfunction; noradrenergic deficiency attention disorder; and serotoninergic deficiency may be associated with affective disorder.

Clinically, PD-D is characterized by insidious onset and slowly progressive dementia. Disturbances in attention and visual-spatial functions along with marked executive dysfunction and moderately impaired memory are characteristic features of PD-D. Cognitive impairment may not be detected in advanced stage PD patients due to the severity of motor findings. In the mental state examination, complex attention and impairment in psychomotor speed are the earliest features detected. The working group formed by the Movement Disorders Society in 2007 published the diagnostic criteria for PD-D (Emre 2007).

Secondary Forms of Dementia (Non-Neurodegenerative)

Vascular Dementia

Vascular dementia (VaD) is a different dementia group in terms of both clinical course and pathogenesis in which cerebral vascular factors play a role in its pathophysiological mechanism. VaD can be classified according to the characteristics of affected vessels, location of the lesion (cortical-subcortical), number of lesions, temporal relationship with stroke (post-stroke or non-stroke), tissue damage type (ischemic, hemorrhagic, or hypoxic-ischemic), course type (stable course after sudden onset or progressive), and presence or absence of other degenerative pathologies. In patients with VaD, genetic inheritance is rare. There is a mutation in the Notch 3 gene on chromosome 19 in CADASIL and in the APP gene on chromosome 21 in Abeta amyloid angiopathy. Fabry disease and hereditary multi-infarct dementia syndrome are other examples of hereditary VaD. Cerebral infarcts, vascular leukoencephalopathy, subcortical lacunar infarcts with vascular leukoencephalopathy, cerebral hemorrhages, and cerebral amyloid angiopathy are the causes of the pathophysiology of VaD (Bingöl 2013).

Since VaD is a heterogeneous group of diseases with many subtypes, it is not possible to talk about a uniform clinical picture. VaD can be examined as the "pre-dementia stage" and "dementia stage" in which dementia is not yet as evident as in degenerative dementias.

Vascular depression occurs in up to 20 percent of VaD patients and can lead to dementia. It is a major depression picture with apathy and psychomotor slowing in the foreground and is resistant to antidepressant treatment. The term *vascular cognitive impairment* such as seen in the MCI stage in the course of degenerative dementias has been suggested in some VaD patients before the manifestation of overt dementia, but diagnostic criteria for vascular cognitive impairment are not yet available. Vascular depression and vascular cognitive impairment are mostly seen in subcortical VaDs. Most post-stroke VaDs are of the ischemic type. In these patients, dementia is expected to begin with whatever the cognitive function of the area affected by the infarct was, and executive dysfunction will be added within months. Post-stroke VaD can develop in up to 25 percent of stroke cases (Bingöl 2013).

Normal Pressure Hydrocephalus

Normal pressure hydrocephalus (NPH) is characterized by enlarged cerebral ventricles (ventriculomegaly), dementia, gait apraxia, and urinary incontinence. NPH is also a potentially reversible syndrome and may be idiopathic or secondary to conditions that block the flow of cerebrospinal fluid (meningitis or subarachnoid hemorrhage) (Graff-Radford 2019).

NPH usually develops within weeks to months, and gait disturbance is often the initial sign. Gait disturbance is typically in the form of gait apraxia. It is characterized by difficulty initiating walking despite the absence of ataxia, instability while standing (magnetic or glue-footed gait). Urinary incontinence occurs later, and patients may not be aware of it. Dementia often has a mild and insidious onset. It is characterized by mental slowing and apathy in the beginning and then global cognitive dysfunction. Other types of dementia such as AD, Parkinsonism, and vascular dementia should be considered in the differential diagnosis.

For the diagnosis of NPH, enlarged lateral ventricles should be seen in neuroimaging with CT or MRI without increasing the prominence of cortical grooves. Ventricular dilation is assessed by the Evans ratio, which is the ratio of the widest frontal horn opening to the largest diameter of the brain in the same axial image. If the Evans ratio is above 0.3, the ratio indicates large ventricles; if it is above 0.33, the ratio indicates large ventricles but is not specific for NPH (Williams 2016). Temporary improvements in walking, cognitive examination, or sphincter functions following 30–50 ml cerebrospinal fluid (CSF) withdrawal by lumbar puncture (tap test) indicate that shunting will be beneficial. Approximately half of the patients show long-term recovery after shunting in idiopathic NPHs (Williams 2016).

Metabolic Causes of Dementia

Chronic renal failure, hyper or hypoparathyroidism, chronic alcoholism, and chronic hypoxic conditions such as COPD, Cushing syndrome, and malnutrition can lead to cognitive disorders and dementia (Gale 2018).

Autoimmune Causes of Dementia

Syndromes with immunological mechanisms have the potential to affect all parts of the central and peripheral nervous system. Distinctive features include acute or subacute onset, rapid progression, signs of inflammation in serum or CSF, and the formation of pathogenic antibodies (Tüzün 2007).

In limbic encephalitis (LE), there is involvement of limbic structures. It can be isolated or occur as a part of paraneoplastic encephalitis or encephalomyelitis. The main features of LE are memory loss, epileptic seizures and behavioral changes, confusional state, irritability, depression, sleep problems, hallucinations, and psychosis. Cranial MRI, EEG, and CSF examinations should be performed in patients with suspected LE (Budhram

2019). On cranial MRI, unilateral or bilateral medial temporal hyperintensity is observed in T2 and flair sections. Lesions rarely contrast enhancement. In cases where cranial MRI examination is normal, FDG-PET examination may show hypometabolism in the temporal lobes. PET examination is also an important and necessary examination because of the possibility of detecting tumor focus in any part of the body. EEG examination shows unilateral or bilateral temporal epileptic activity and focal or diffuse slow-wave activity. CSF examination, lymphocyte predominant pleocytosis and increased protein are detected. The glucose level is usually normal. As an exception, CSF examination is normal in limbic encephalitis associated with the voltage-gated potassium channel antibody (Tüzün 2007). Most cases of paraneoplastic limbic encephalitis are lost due to progressive neurological destruction and/or cancer-related causes. Paraneoplastic LE is most commonly associated with small cell lung cancer, and symptoms typically precede the diagnosis of the underlying cancer (Tüzün 2007).

Infectious Causes of Dementia

Infections that lead to cognitive impairment and dementia syndrome primarily include HIV, syphilis, herpes simplex and other viruses, encephalitis, and chronic meningitis (Tuncer 2013).

HIV causes a chronic neurodegenerative process with cognitive, motor, and behavioral symptoms. Cognitive involvement shows that the characteristics of subcortical dementia, behavioral changes, and apathy accompanying mental-motor slowing are the main features. Attention, concentration, psychomotor speed, memory, learning, planning in executive functions, abstraction, and inhibition of inappropriate responses are the frequently affected areas. Cognitive changes are accompanied by symmetrical motor signs and slowness. Cortical atrophy and white matter changes are detected in cranial MRI imaging. Cryptococcal meningitis can mimic HIV-related dementia, so cryptococcal antigen should be checked in the CSF examination for differential diagnosis. Cytomegalovirus encephalitis and neurosyphilis are diseases that should be considered in differential diagnosis.

Syphilis is a chronic, bacterial infection caused by *Treponema pallidum*. It is frequently sexually transmitted. Dementia, focal neurological deficits, and psychiatric symptoms such as paranoia, mania, psychosis, delirium, and personality and mood changes can be seen together.

Lyme disease is a systemic disease caused by *Borrelia burgdorferi*. It is transmitted through a tick bite. Cranial nerve involvement, meningitis, polyradiculopathy, depression, psychosis, and dementia may be seen in neuroborreliosis. Since it is a treatable disease, early diagnosis is important.

Herpes simplex virus (HSV) encephalitis is the most common fatal sporadic encephalitis. Except for a few rare cases, HSV encephalitis is caused by HSV-1. Cranial involvement is in the temporal lobes and is usually symmetrical. Clinical findings include acute and subacute onset headache, fever, behavioral change, cognitive deterioration (memory and language impairment), and focal and generalized seizures. Widespread background slow-wave activity and periodic epileptiform activity in the temporal lobes are characteristic EEG findings. Herpes virus DNA can be detected by the polymerase chain reaction method. In doubtful cases, it is important to start acyclovir treatment without delay.

Subacute sclerosing panencephalitis is a chronic disease caused by the measles virus that is common in children but can also occur in adults. Progressive dementia, focal and generalized seizures, myoclonus, ataxia, rigidity, and visual disturbances are clinical findings.

Progressive multifocal leukoencephalopathy is an infection caused by JC papovaviruses in immunocompromised patients and progresses with rapidly progressive dementia and focal neurological symptoms (Tuncer 2013).

Case 1

A 70-year-old woman who is a secondary school graduate, a widow, and childless died six months ago due to cardiac reasons. Due to the dispute of her heirs, the court decision was appealed. One of her sibling's two children took care of her, as she was treated for heart failure and needed physical support. Due to her depressive mood and the inability to be alone, a caregiver was found first, then the younger nephew took her into his own home and took care of her. At that time, she was able to do her own work at home, but she needed support in the bathroom and regular treatments due to shortness of breath, and she was able to maintain her other self-care routines. Sometimes she forgot names and recent events. She knew her relatives and assets and could track her salary, and her social judgment was good, but she often had hospital admissions due to palpitations, shortness of breath, swelling of the legs, and high blood pressure. When she applied to the hospital for a cardiac examination about a year ago, due to her forgetfulness, the geriatrician started to treat her with the drugs used in the treatment of AD. A diagnosis of dementia was written, and a medication report was issued so that the patient's nephew could help her take the medication more easily. However, detailed memory and mental functions were not evaluated and recorded. The patient had a level of forgetfulness that did not affect her life, which was described by her relative with whom she lived. Care support was required not because of mental state disorders but because of her physical diseases. Five months before she died, she decided to give her house to her nephew who took care of her. When she was told that a medical report was needed for this procedure, she was examined by a psychiatrist, and a report was given stating that her mental functions were compatible with her age, and she proceeded to donate her house to her nephew. After the death of the patient, her other nephew sued the younger nephew on the grounds that his aunt was treated for the diagnosis of AD. He declared that his aunt was deceived, she could take care of herself and was not well cared for by the nephew, and even though her house was donated, she did not have the mental strength and legal capacity to make the decision. In this case, as an expert, we were assigned as an arbitrator in relation to whether the patient had dementia in the year before her death (when she donated her assets) and whether the nephew had legal capacity at that time.

Discussion

- With the available data, what will we pay attention to when making a decision for the patient who has died?
- Discuss how the records of the patient are particularly important.
- Not all forgetfulness is dementia. Do you believe that subjective cognitive impairment and mild cognitive impairment cases are not dementia and that patients with these conditions can make their own decisions?
- AD treatment, whose benefit has not yet been proven, was started for this patient. Was the diagnosis of dementia misleading in court evidence?
- Detailed cognitive tests should have been conducted. Was it appropriate for the physician who saw the patient once, instead of her regular physician and the committee, to make the decisions about the patient?

Case 2

A 68-year-old female patient, a housewife, lives with her assistant. She came to clinic with her lawyer and son. In her history, it was learned that she was frequently diagnosed with depression for many years and was hospitalized three times in a mental and neurological diseases hospital. Her past medical history includes obesity, hypertension, and diabetes mellitus. The patient, who divorced her husband many years ago, has two sons living in the United States in the same city. She was diagnosed with bipolar disorder during her psychiatric hospitalizations. The elder son of the patient filed a lawsuit with the claim that his mother did not have the legal capacity and was not able to make the decision that her assets could be taken by his brother under these conditions. The patient was cognitively healthy, and a health board report was conducted when she transferred her assets to her younger son. Her son and lawyer say that she needs help because of obesity and rheumatic disease. Her lawyer reports that the patient did not have dementia and that she had a lot of trouble and depression due to her past marriage. A mental assessment was not done. In the cognitive examination of the patient, she appeared conscious and cooperative, her place and person orientation was intact, she had time disorientation, and her memory was preserved but she could not recall. The doctors detected problems with understanding proverbial meanings, impaired judgment, some loss of insight, planning disorders, and attention disorder. She did not have a depressive mood, but her affect was dull. When asked about her assets, she could not say exactly what she had and stated that she gave some of her property to both of her sons (whereas she only gave it to her younger son).

Discussion

- Dementia is seen at a higher rate in chronic psychiatric diseases (schizophrenia, bipolar disorder, etc.). Therefore, should patients with such diagnoses be evaluated before important decisions need to be made?
- Dementia may not be very visible, as memory defects are not in the foreground as in AD. Judgment disorder, rather than executive dysfunction, may affect the decision-making process. Can the family can use this situation to make a decision?
- What is the importance of detailed interviews, a detailed cognitive evaluation of the patient, and the views of the psychiatrist who followed up with her?
- Should how much information the patient has about the subject, her opinion on the subject, whether she remembers that she made a commitment, and whether she was forced by someone else to make this decision be questioned and recorded in the individual interview?

CONCLUSION

When a patient is evaluated with a complaint of forgetfulness, a detailed mental examination, cognitive tests, and imaging and laboratory tests should be performed. To protect patients and their relatives, any diagnoses and decisions made from the examinations should be recorded.

REFERENCES

Arvanitakis, Z. Shah, RC. Bennett, DA. (2019) Diagnosis and Management of Dementia: Review, *J JAMA*, Volume 322, Number 16, p: 1589-1599.

Barrett, AM. Wolf, S. Reischies, FM. et al. (2005), Unawareness of cognitive deficit (cognitive anosognosia) in probable AD and control subjects. *Neurology*, 64:693-699.

Bingöl, A.(2013) *Vasculer Dementia. Neurology Essential Book*. Emre, M. editor, Part: 5. Gunes Medical Bookstore 1st ed. Ankara p984-993).

Brown, RG. Lacomblez, L. Landwehrmeyer, BG. et al. (2010) Cognitive impairment in patients with multiple system atrophy and progressive supranuclear palsy. *Brain,* 133:2382–2393.

Budhram, A. Leung, A. Nicolle, MW. Burneo, JG (2019), Diagnosing autoimmune limbic encephalitis, *CMAJ*, May 13;191:E529-34.

Crutch, SJ. Schott, JM. Rabinovici, GD. et al. (2017) Alzheimer's Assosiation ISTAART Atypical Alzheimer's Disease and Associated Syndromes Professional Interest Area, Consensus Classification of Posterior Cortical Atrophy. *Alzheimer's Dement*, 13:870-884).

Emre, M. (2013) *Alzheimer's Disease, Neurology Essential Book*. Emre, M. editor, Part:5. Gunes Medical Bookstore 1st ed. Ankara p: 955-962.

Emre, M. (2007) Clinical features, pathophysiology and treatment of dementia associated with Parkinson's Disease. *Handbook of Clinical Neurology*, 83:401-419.

Emre, M. Aarsland, D. Brown, R. Burn, DJ. et al. (2007) Clinical Diagnostic Criteria for Dementia Associated with Parkinson's Disease, *Movement Disorders*, Vol. 22, No. 12, p:1689-1707.

Gale, SA. Acar, D. Daffner, KR. (2018), Dementia, *The American Journal of Medicine* https://doi.org/10.1016/j.amjmed.2018.01.022.

Graff-Radford, NR. Jones, D. (2019) *Normal pressure hydrocephalus, Continuum (Minneap Minn)*, 25(1, Dementia):165–186.

Hanağası, H. (2013) Lewy Body Dementia, Neurology Essential Book. Emre, M. editor, *Dementia Part: 5*. Gunes Medical Bookstore 1st ed. p: 974-978.

Hanson, JC. Lippa, CF. (2009) Lewy body dementia. *International Review of Neurobiology*, 84:215-228.

Lobotesis, K. Fenwick, JD. Phipps, A. et al. (2001) Occipital hypoperfusion on SPECT in dementia with Lewy bodies but not AD, *Neurology*, 56:643-649.

McKhann, G. Drachman, D. Folstein, M. et al. (1984) Report of the NINCDS-ADRDA work group under the auspices of department of health and human service task force on Alzheimer's Disease. *Neurology*, 34:939-944.

McKeith, I. (2004) Dementia with Lewy bodies and other difficult diagnosis *Int Psychogeriatr,* 16:123-127.

McKeith, I. Dickson, D. Lowe, J. et al. (2005) Diagnosis and management of dementia with Lewy bodies. *Neurology*, 65:1863–72.

Mesulam, M. Wicklund, A. Johnson, N. et al. (2008) Alzheimer and frontotemporal pathology in subsets of primary progressive aphasia. *Annals of Neurology,* 63:709-719.

Miller, B. Llibre Guerra, JJ. (2019) Frontotemporal dementia, *Handb Clin Neurol,* 165:33-45.

Nasreddine, ZS. Phillips, NA. B. dirian, V. et al. (2005) The Montreal Cognitive Assessment, MoCA: a brief screening tool for mild cognitive impairment. *J Am Geriatr Soc*, 53(4):695-699.

Parakh, R. Roy, E. Koo, E. Black, S. (2004), Pantomime and imitation of limb gestures in relation to the severity of Alzheimer's Disease. *Brain Cogn,* 55:272.

Peters, F. Collette, F. Degueldre, C. et al. (2009), The neural correlates of verbal short-term memory in Alzheimer's Disease: an fMRI study. *Brain*, 132:1833-1846.

Ridgwa, GR. Lehmann, M. Barnes, J et al. (2012) Early onset Alzheimer disease clinical variants: multivariate analyses of cortical thickness. *Neurology*, 79: 80-84.

Salem, LC. Vogel, A. Ebstrup, J. Linneberg, A. Waldemar, G. (2015) Subjective cognitive complaints included in diagnostic evaluation of dementia helps accurate diagnosis in a mixed memory clinic cohort. Int *J Geriatr Psychiatry,* 30(12):1177-118.

Scheltens, P. Blennow, K. Breteler, MB. et al. (2016), Alzheimer's disease *Lancet,* 388:505–17.

Sivasathiaseelan, H. Marshall, CR. Agustus, JL. (2019)Frontotemporal Dementia: A Clinical Review, *Semin Neurol,* 39:251–263.

Tuncer, N. (2013), Infectious causes of Dementia, Emre M, editor, *Neurology Essential Book.* Part: 5. Gunes Medical Bookstore 1st ed. Ankara p993-997.

Tüzün, E. Dalmau, J. (2007), Limbic encephalitis and variants: classification, diagnosis and treatment. *Neurologist,* 13:261-271.

Wenning, GK. Geser, F. (2007) Multiple system atrophy. Jankoviç J. Tolosa E, editors. *Parkinson's Disease & Movement Disorders.* Chap: 6 Philadelphia: Lippincott Williams&Wilkins, 5th ed. p.175-185.

Williams, M. A. Malm, J. (2016) *Diagnosis and Treatment of Idiopathic Normal Pressure Hydrocephalus, Continuum (Minneap Minn),* 22(2):579–599.

Yo-el S, J. Lucey, BP. Holtzman, DM. (2014) Sleep and Alzheimer's Disease -a bidirectional relationship. *Nature reviews Neurology,* 10:115).

In: Forensic Psychiatry …
Editor: Nursen Turan Yurtsever
ISBN: 978-1-53619-530-9

Chapter 9

CHILD CUSTODY EVALUATIONS

Elif Akin[1,*] and Aliye Tugba Bahadir[2]
[1]Izmir Democracy University Buca Seyfi Demirsoy Training and Research Hospital, Child and and Adolescent Psychiatry Clinic, Izmir, Turkey
[2]Marmara University School of Medicine, Department of Child and Adolescent Psychiatry, Istanbul, Turkey

ABSTRACT

Divorce rates are increasing year after year worldwide. A significant number of divorces involve custody litigation, and thousands of children are caught in the middle of the often-protracted legal battles that occur between parents. A forensic evaluation in a child custody case is a comprehensive process requiring the abilities of a therapist who has knowledge of some ethical issues. For a complete child custody evaluation, it is crucial to interview the child and adults and obtain information from other family members and related people. In deciding the best interests of the child, evaluators should be aware of the developmental processes of the child and the parental issues, and they must do this in an objective and sensible environment and declare their expert opinion to the court at the

* Corresponding Author's E-mail: elif_akin@yahoo.com.

end of the evaluation. The presence of special issues such as sexual abuse or parental alienation allegations may complicate the evaluation process and require specialized assessments. Some psychological instruments are also used to gain information. Evaluators are required to assess factors related to the best interests of the child.

A report written objectively from a child-focused perspective contributes to judicial decision-making at its best.

INTRODUCTION

Divorce rates are increasing year after year worldwide. Around the world between 1970 and 2008, the number of divorces has increased. The rates have even doubled from 2.6 to 5.5 divorces for every 1,000 married people (OECD; United Nations 2019). Since litigation over custody or visitation occurs in about 10 percent of divorces, approximately 100,000 children a year stay between the parents during this compelling divorce process (Bernet 2002).

Divorce, in terms of law, is defined as the ending of a marriage contract between partners. However, this process is not as simple as its definition implies because it affects all family members and the subjects they are in close contact with. In addition, if the couples have a common child or children, the divorce goes beyond a process that occurs between the couple. When this process is not managed in a healthy manner by the parents, children are often the ones who are most affected.

International legal arrangements such as the United Nations Convention on the Rights of a Child and a country's own laws ensure that children live and complete their development in a safe and comfortable environment. The United Nations Convention on the Rights of a Child emphasizes that the mother and father are responsible for the child's upbringing and development and that a child must grow in a happy, loving, and sensible environment in order to develop a complete and compatible personality.

During the divorce process, the rights and responsibilities of the parents must be reconstructed based on the best interests of the child. Their values on parenting, their plans about what the child needs in the future, their ability to present a regular and loving environment to the child, and their inappropriate or abusive behaviors, which could have a negative effect on the child, must be considered (APA 1995). If parents disagree about this new arrangement, family courts must determine which parent will take custody of the child and, after assessing the reports of the experts and professionals, what the relationship of both parents will be with the child. In some high-conflict divorce proceedings, family courts ask for opinions from the mental health professionals about some issues, including determination of custody, changing of custody, and arrangements of the relationship between the child and parent (adjustment, changing, or interruption of the visitation pattern). At this time in child and adolescent psychiatry clinics, interviews are made separately with both the child and parents. When necessary, all family members are involved, and appropriate psychiatric assessment scales and techniques are used and adult psychiatry consultation is warranted for the assessment of the mental health of the parents. Additionally, when needed, visits to the home and school are made, and the living conditions and social environment of the child and parents are investigated. An opinion report arranged by a judicial committee is then presented to the court. In a high-conflict divorce proceeding, assessments and decisions made by professionals are important in minimizing the effect of the process on the child's development.

Mental health professionals are included in custody and visitation decisions in several different ways (Bernet 2002). It is commonly seen that a child might have been and still may be on psychotherapy when the parents decide to divorce and the process begins. In this circumstance, the therapist aims at helping the family handle the situation and cope with the problems they encounter during this process (Garner 1991). Another situation can be that the court may want a child to be assessed in order to determine the need for therapy as a result or part of its custody decree. Here, too, rather than influence the result of the legal dispute, the therapist tries to help the child adapt to what the judge decides and contracts well-established contact with the mother and father. This makes those in this difficult and argumentative situation—which commonly occurs in custody disputes—more prone to reaching an agreement between the parties (Marlow and Sauber 1990;

Saposnek 1998). The therapist may also take a role as a guide for both the parents, aiding the parents with the joint common aim of being cooperative to do the best for their children (Barnum 1987). If the mother or the father has an emotional disorder warranting treatment, then the therapist might help in this instance. Finally, the mental health professional may be involved for the assessment of the custody and visitation program.

These assessments require a psychiatric and/or psychological evaluation of the child, the mother, and the father, and recommendations must be made in the best interests of the child. In custody litigations, the mental health professional is referred as a consultant to the court or as a professional to assess the parents if needed (Bernet 2002).

IMPACT OF DIVORCE

The divorce process can be a compelling adjustment period for children, especially when parents cannot manage the process in a healthy manner. Therefore, conflict between parents may be the most critical factor in the adjustment of children in divorcing families. Children are vulnerable and tend to develop emotional problems when they are in the middle of the battle between their parents, and they may feel stuck and not know what to do when they feel insecure. This situation may cause significant emotional and behavioral problems such as sadness, anger, worry about themselves and their family, and aggressive behavior. These problems more commonly occur after two years. After separation, children are often fearful and stressed due to the disruption of family integrity and change in their routines, living conditions, and facilities; are often scared about being abandoned or alone and might feel insecure or sometimes; might blame themselves when they are caught in a battle between both parents. The forensic evaluator must be conscious of these emotional and behavioral effects of divorce on children because they can secondarily affect the child's statements and responses (Lubit 2005).

Another important issue is that many children feel like they must do something to correct the situation, and even though they are unable to manage the situation, they may act like a mediator between the two hostile parents. When children take this role, they can be damaged in many ways. Their relationship with their own parents may be negatively affected, and this can also negatively influence their adult relationships in the future. Perhaps the biggest effect of divorce occurs when children grow up and try to maintain their own relationships. Because they do not have a healthy managed inner model for lasting adult relationships, they are at risk of having problems in family and marital relationships (Lubit 2005).

Essential Aspects of Development

The essentials of child development are important to understand since the arrangements of placement and visitation should be made after considering children's needs after a divorce. First, how young children perceive time differs from adults. Time is seen as progressing more slowly for children. So, when designing visitation schedules, especially overnight visits and vacation times, children's different experiences with time must be kept in mind.

It is important to remember that preschool and kindergarten children's lives may be mostly focused on home. As children move into school age and adolescence, their environment expands to the social community, and friends gain importance in the children's lives. Living arrangements should be made regarding normal developmental experiences of childhood to allow the children to achieve specific skills and interests.

To develop a healthy coherent identity, children and adolescents need to internalize positive images of and morals from their parents. If one parent behaves in an inappropriate manner, it should be determined if the child is affected negatively.

During the stormy divorce process, outside support has powerful importance as a source of security and stability in children's lives. These sources include religion, ties to friends, adults in the community, and the sibling relationships. Maintaining these ties should be part of the custody decision (Lubit 2005).

Crucial questions include: Which parent can best support the children's development? Which parent best provides support and encourages the children to learn new skills? Which parent can best help the children deal with anxiety-provoking situations and provide them with emotional sustenance, support, and encouragement to engage them in developing new skills? Which parent is best able to help the children learn to think about new situations, develop trust in themselves, and validate their feelings? Does one of the parents fail to protect the children adequately from dangers in the community or from their own mistakes? Which parent provides more assistance and encouragement with schoolwork and learning opportunities outside of school? Which parent can better guide the children to learn social skills? Does one of the parents invalidate the children's emotional experiences? Which parent is better able to assess the children's abilities and emotional needs accurately and adjust their parenting style to fit the developmental needs of the children? Children's fantasies are a large part of growing up. How each parent is able to help the children with fantasies is an important part of parenting and something that should be assessed in the custody evaluation. It is also important to figure out which parent can best support the children's fantasy attachments or admiration of a powerful, admirable figure and which one responds with jealousy or belittling of the children's attachment to an outside hero (Lubit 2005).

To make decisions about the best parenting choice, the clinician needs to assess the ability of parents to be aware of and respond to the children's specific needs and temperaments. In courts, when determining who will get custody of the children, evaluations that use scales are needed to assess parenting skills; parents' abilities, deficiencies, and values; their past parenting experiences and involvement in raising the child; their past medical history; and the capacity of the parent to recognize and respond to the children's needs. But, in some circumstances when the mental health status of a parent is in question or is inadequate, mental health professionals are asked for their opinion.

CHILD CUSTODY

An evaluation made by a mental health professional in custody cases may be indicated in the following situations (Kraus and Thomas 2011): (1) when parenting abilities are affected by the presence of a mental disorder in one or both parents; (2) when the child has a mental disorder; (3) when violence in the family (including abuse by a parent, sibling, or the child) has been documented; and (4) when parental alienation of a noncustodial parent has been detected.

A forensic evaluator needs to present the results of an evaluation as an expert (Chung et al. 2020). Two features are important: first, the evaluator must have no therapeutic relationship with the subject, and second, confidentiality has some limits in a forensic evaluation.

The order of the evaluation may show variability and must contain the following parent-, child-, and family-related factors (Kraus and Thomas 2011): (1) parent-related: parenting skills, physical and mental health, substance abuse, current and previous involvement in the child welfare facilities, and willingness to cooperate with the other parent in the raising child; (2) child-related: mental health, attachment to each parent, and preferences regarding custody or living arrangements; and (3) family-related: history of domestic violence, allegations of abuse, and allegations of parental alienation.

The Process of Evaluation

In conducting a complete custody evaluation, it is best if the evaluator communicates with all members of the family. Parents, stepparents, and all the children should be interviewed for a complete evaluation. The evaluator may want to interview other significant individuals, such as the current love interest of either parent, grandparents, the babysitters, school personnel, and the psychotherapists, either in person or by phone (Bernet 1983).

The overall evaluation process includes three areas: interviews with and evaluations of the parents, interview with and evaluation of the child (including of parent-child interactions in preschoolers), and collateral information gathering (Bow and Quinell 2002).

Interview with Parents (Parental Assessment)

Because this is a forensic evaluation and not a therapeutic interview, parents should be informed that the interviews are not privileged and that a report collected from the information in the interviews will be written and presented to the court.

The parents should be interviewed about the following items: (1) the chronology of the parents' marriage, including childbirth, separation, and divorce; (2) the current status of legal proceedings; (3) court orders regarding the custody evaluation; (4) the current visitation schedule and custody status; (5) each parent's perception of his or her own relationship with the child; (6) each parent's understanding of his or her child and response to the child's specific needs; (7) each parent's parenting plan if granted custody; and (8) each parent's personal history, criminal record, family history, social support system, and history of psychiatric treatment (Chung et al. 2020).

It is often helpful to have an initial meeting with the mother and father, which enables them to clarify the aim, content, and structure of the custody evaluation. Interviewing and testing as a part of evaluation are programmed in this initial conference. It also enables the evaluator to gather information not just from both parents but also from pediatricians, teachers, therapists, and other related individuals. Ultimately, an initial meeting will allow the evaluator to see the attitudes of parents and how they react to each other and whether they are willing to agree to a solution (Bernet 2002).

The evaluator interviews each parent separately and evaluates each parent's abilities and behaviors. This evaluation may require one long meeting of two to three hours or several shorter meetings (Bernet 2002).

During the interviews with each parent, the evaluator should determine what the parent focuses on most—the child or the other parent. Many parents argue and complain and thus move away from the most important issue. In these conditions, the evaluator must warn the parent about the time and program and that wasting time would not be in the child's best interests (Chung et al. 2020). The evaluator should also determine the child's developmental history and usual routine (Herman 1997). Ultimately, to evaluate the parents' behaviors and perspectives about caring for the child as a parent, the evaluator should learn what the parents will do with their child and how they will spend time with the child in every situation whether or not they are granted custody. They will also need to evaluate their responses to questions such as "If you are granted custody, how will you help your child maintain a good relationship with your ex-spouse?" and "If you are not granted custody, how will you maintain a good relationship with your child?" (Herman 1997). The evaluator not only assesses the content of the answers but also observes the parents' attitudes toward the aim of the interview and the parents' contact patterns with the evaluator (Bernet 2002).

To evaluate the parents' parenting patterns, the evaluator should determine how parents will spend time with the child and what changes will occur in the relationship between the child and parent after the result of the custody case (Chung et al. 2020). The evaluation may also include questions about each parent's practice and philosophy of parental discipline (Herman 1997). Assessment of each parent's caretaking history (especially, which parent is more involved in feeding, bathing, supervising homework, organizing birthday parties, and taking the child to the pediatrician) is crucial. The more involved parent is more likely to be granted custody (Bernet 2002).

The following significant issues should be considered as part of the custody evaluation (Herman 1997): (1) the child's and each parent's wishes or preferences regarding custody; (2) the child's interactions with each parent, siblings, and individuals who may significantly influence the child; (3) the child's adjustment to home, school, and community environments; (4) the physical and mental health of all individuals involved; (5) parental attempts at alienation; (6) the quality and nature of the emotional relationship between each parent and the child; (7) each parent's emotional and psychological stability; (8) each parent's parenting skills; (9) each parent's openness to visitation by the other parent; (10) each parent's proposals for the child's custody and visitation arrangements; (11) each parent's pre-divorce parental role and parenting capacity; (12) each parent's degree of anger and distress related to the divorce; and (13) each parent's sexual orientation.

It is important to evaluate the understanding of each parent's ability to understand the child and the child's needs and his or her ability to appropriately respond to those needs. For this reason, the parents should be questioned about the child in detail, including the following topics: (1) the strengths of child: what the child likes and wants for the future and each parent's attitude toward those wishes; (2) the needs of the child: frequency, intensity, duration of problematic behaviors, and the way the parents deal with the behavior; (3) the traumas and stresses the child has had; (4) the child's developmental history: who has taken care of which needs of the child in the past—buying clothing, taking to school, cooking, arranging play dates, taking to the pediatrician, helping with homework, bathing, and talking to teachers; (5) the concerns about the other parent's relationship with and caretaking of the child; and (6) the response to any allegations by the other parent.

To evaluate which parent will provide the child with the best developmental experiences, parents should be asked about the following items (Lubit 2005): (1) contact with the other parent; (2) schooling; (3) contact with relatives; (4) recreational activities; (5) socialization with other children; (6) religious activities; (7) special needs; and (8) emotional stress about the divorce.

To determine which parent is more stable and has the better emotional balance and intellectual ability to provide the child with the structure, emotional support, and role model needed to grow into a capable adult, the following items should be examined in the parent history (Lubit 2005): (1) parents' family of origin, education, work history, history of relationships, current relationship, cultural/religious ties, and family ties; (2) history of prior marriages, if any; (3) children from prior marriages, those custody relationships, and how those relationships will affect the children from the current marriage; (4) history of psychological/substance abuse problems and treatment, medical history, and legal history; (5) use of alcohol and other drugs; (6) parents' beliefs about discipline and how they will support the child; (7) parents' ability to be aware of the child's needs; (8) feelings about the child having contact with the other parent; (9) extended family with whom they want the child to have contact; (10) family psychiatric and medical problems; and (11) whether the child reminds the parent of someone and if the parent identifies with the child.

Child custody evaluators should also gather information about parental thoughts on the current family situation. Topics for exploration include the following items (Lubit 2005): (1) history of the relationship, including reason for the divorce; (2) current living situation; (3) current visitation arrangements and problems with the arrangement; (4) why the parents feel they would be the better custodial parent; (5) concerns about the other parent having custody; (6) beliefs about the other parent's concerns about them; (7) ability to identify and acknowledge one's own weakness and shortcomings; and (8) ability to appreciate mental or physical health problems the child has or might develop and willingness to cooperate with physicians or clinicians in evaluation and treatment.

Interview with the Child

An interview with the child plays an important and integrative role in custody evaluation. The meetings with the child should be done to accomplish a clinical assessment of the child, evaluate the attachment of the child to each parent, and clarify how the child was influenced by the divorce or separation and assess whether the child has been indoctrinated in some way. Mostly, the evaluator should assess which parent the child prefers and what the child wants in terms of custody and visitation and determine his or her causes for that preference. In several situations, however, such as where the child does not have enough mental capacity to choose or when the child could be confused, this may be inappropriate (Bernet 2002).

Interviews with the child should consist of at least two meetings where each parent joins the child. How the interview is done and what will be included could change in relation to the child's best interests (Bernet 2002).

The parents should be instructed to tell their children that an evaluator will be meeting with the family to make recommendations on how they can best take care of the children now that they are living apart (Lubit 2005). The evaluators should interview each child, except for infants, and be careful about each child's needs regarding his or her developmental period and age. If the child has enough maturity to express his or her opinion, the evaluator should evaluate the child's expressions about what she or he wants. In a written report to the court, the evaluator should relate the obtained information about the child's thoughts and emotions and give the importance of these thoughts and feelings (Martingale et al. 2007). As mentioned before, when evaluating the child, the evaluator must consider clinical diagnoses, level of attachment to each parent, any expressed preferences for either parent, and any evidence of indoctrination by either parent. Siblings should be interviewed and observed when they are side by side to evaluate how they interact and how supportive they are with each other (Chung et al. 2020).

When interviewing the child, the evaluator should begin by telling the child the aim of the meeting and the evaluator's task in the proceeding. Children as young as 3 years, who know what the judge does, might have the capacity to find out the task of the evaluator (Herman 1997). The evaluator may then continue asking questions to learn about what is in the child's mind concerning the family's current and future situation. To communicate with the child in an environment where the child will feel safe and comfortable, suitable methods should be used according to the child's age. To communicate with and understand what is happening inside of younger children, toys and play compatible with the interests of their age can be useful to the evaluator (Herman 1997). If they can be in a room without a parent, children as young as three can usually be interviewed alone. The evaluator should be careful about asking the children, especially young children, where they would prefer to live. If the child declares which parent she or he wants to live with, the evaluator should question the child and learn the details about the child's choice (Chung et al. 2020). Questions should be asked and presented in a natural way without exacerbation. It can ease the child's mind to tell him or her that the final decision will be made by the judge, not the child or the evaluator (Bernet 2002). After five years of age, especially for adolescents, what the child thinks and wants is considered much more important. When a child or adolescent is considered developmentally mature and can declare his or her own thoughts, his or her wants and preferences must be evaluated much more seriously (Martindale et al. 2007).

Interviews with preschool-aged children may begin with the parent and the child together. Regarding infants, the evaluator should observe the attachment relationship between the parent and the child and look for the parent's suitable actions for the child's needs regarding the child's developmental period. The evaluator should give a task to the parent in which he or she spends time with the child, maybe a playing activity or doing something outside. This could give the evaluator a chance to observe how the child and the parent react to each other and what they experience. Assessments of the reactions and relationship between the parent and child are significant (AFCC 1994). If the evaluator cannot retrieve information about parent-child observations, he or she should declare the reason (AAML 2013). However, the task given by the evaluator should be something the parent and the child prefer, and the play should be started by the child (Bernet 2002), or the evaluator could direct a parent and child of appropriate age to cooperatively complete a task. The evaluator should observe how the interaction between the parent and the child affects the child and if the parent comforts the child (Herman 1997). About halfway through the interview, the parent should be asked to leave the room, and the evaluator should tell the child that the parent will be out of the room but will reunite with the child whenever she or he feels uncomfortable. When the parent leaves the room, the evaluator should observe how the child reacts and how the parents manage this. The evaluator should continue to communicate with the child according to his or her age and interests, which could entail playing or drawing with younger children. Finally, the evaluator should assess both the child and parent when they reunite (Bernet 2002).

In an interview with school-aged children, the techniques for the clinical evaluation of children can be used. The child may mention issues such as school, peers, activities they like to do, and family relationships. Projective questions can be asked, and projective tests, including stories or pictures, can be used (Bernet 2002).

Drawing is also one way that children express themselves. The evaluator can ask the child to draw a child, person, or family and may want the child to tell a story about what is going on in the drawing. This may give some clues. The evaluator may ask the child to make up a list of negatives and positives of each parent, and this will also present clues about each parent's attitudes and behaviors. The evaluator may also ask the child where she or he wants to live, making sure the child knows that the decision will be made by the judge, not the child or the evaluator (Bernet 2002).

In interviews with adolescents, the evaluator may start by asking them about what they think about the current family situation. This enables the evaluator to learn about the adolescents' thoughts about why they think the parents are separating, how they assess their parents' attitudes both toward them and toward each other during the divorce process, and how they think their lives will be influenced by this situation (Bernet 2002). Most adolescents have both positive and negative thoughts about living with each parent, particular visitation arrangements, and how they can stay out of the battle between the parents and protect their own lives from the negative effects of divorce. Adolescents seem to have mostly clear preferences about custody. In this circumstance, the evaluator should determine the causes (Bernet 2002).

Collateral Informations

Information collected from outside core family members is also important for comparing the information obtained from both sides of the case (Chung et al. 2020). The custody evaluator must be aware that the accuracy of information acquired from the litigants may be limited and may investigate these given oral reports or any other claims by collecting additional information and asking other sources for their statements (Kraus and Thomas 2011). The evaluator, after getting permission from parents, should also collect information from other sources such as stepparents, grandparents, caregivers, siblings, etc. In some cases, getting information from the family's pediatrician by phone can be suitable since he or she can share unbiased observations about the parents. Acquiring information from schoolteachers and daycare workers may also be helpful, but the evaluator must be aware that they might be in close contact with one of the parents. Also, therapists can be another source of information about both the child and parents for the forensic evaluator (Bernet 2002). Collateral information can also be gathered from police reports, the child's or parents' previous or current therapists, and earlier trial hearings (Bernet 2002; Kraus and Thomas 2011). The evaluator must be aware of the significance of collecting data from multiple sources in a comprehensive custody evaluation (Martindale et al. 2007).

Psychological Tests Used in an Evaluation

In child custody evaluations, psychological testing is a way of collecting objective supportive information about the evaluator's thoughts that helps avoid bias and possible faults in clinical interviews and enables the evaluator to test the information collected from other sources (Gould 1998). Most mental health professionals use standard psychological tests in custody evaluations.

A psychological test that is used for custody evaluations must satisfy five criteria (Heilburn 1992): (1) widespread use and universality; (2) evidence of adequate reliability; (3) relevance to the legal issue at hand, established by validation research; (4) standardized administration for generalizability; and (5) consideration of the effects of the response style on the test results (e.g., "faking good," malingering, social desirability). The evaluator should use the psychological test in a standardized form without any changes (Chung et al. 2020).

Comprehensive personality inventories such as the Minnesota Multiphasic Personality Inventory-2 (Butcher et al. 1989) and the Personality Assessment Inventory (Morey 1991) can be used to determine the presence of mental illness in the parents. Information about abuse or undesirable and inappropriate behaviors can be obtained from these tests (Bernet 2002).

In some situations, it may be helpful to perform a formal intellectual test (if there is a doubt about a parent's cognitive abilities) or a battery of projective tests (if there is a question about the diagnosis of a parent's mental illness). Projective psychological tests constitute an opportunity to observe the parent's efforts to cope with an unstructured and stressful situation and provide information about psychological resources and characteristics. Other psychological tests, such as the Parenting Stress Index (Abidin 1995), can provide information about a parent's level of attachment to the child, the perceived problem areas in the child, and the perceived helpfulness of the spouse. The Ackerman-Schoendorf Parent Evaluation of Custody Test (Ackerman and Schoendorf 1994) is designed to assess the fitness of parents for custody. This test is composed of three scales: observational, social, and cognitive-emotional. If psychological testing is used, the same tests should be administered to both parents (Bernet 2002).

In children, the use of psychological tests can be helpful. Behavior rating scales such as the Achenbach Child Behavior Checklist (Achenbach 1991) and the Personality Inventory for Children (Lachar 1999) can define specific traits and problems.

Courtroom Testimony

Sometimes testimony in court is needed. If the evaluator is not familiar with the process in court, it is beneficial to consult an experienced colleague before testifying. The evaluator should bring all the materials to the trial in case they may need to be used for cross-examination (Herman 1997).

Case 1

Meltem is an eight-year-old girl whose mother and father divorced four years ago. Her mother claimed that her father had been sexually abusing her in the visitations of the past six months. Her mother wanted the father to have restrictions on visitation and wanted him to be punished as a result of the claim. The attitude of the mother toward the child psychiatrist and the forensic medicine expert was disturbing. She had an insisting attitude, she wanted to prolong the interviews with inconsistent information, and she brought some of the "evidence" to the assessments of both departments. In the psychiatric assessment of the child, there were no symptoms or signs suggestive of any anxiety disorder or depression; the child stated that she missed her dad. But the mother insisted that Meltem had symptoms related to anxiety. Two separate interviews that were scheduled two weeks apart with the mother revealed inconsistent symptoms related to anxiety. At some point during the play with the child, the child whispered "we are losing time here," and she restated that she missed her dad. In particular, the former expression of the child attracted the attention of the child psychiatrist, and afterwards, a meeting was planned with the forensic medicine department. After the psychiatric consultation of the mother, it turned out that the mother hadborderline personality disorder, antisocial personality traits, and moderate depression, and she herself was sexually abused around the age of seven. The mother was still very angry with the father and blamed him for her loneliness. After a quick decision to get married in the past, they later divorced due to an ongoing severe conflict that emerged after the third month of their marriage. The father was shocked to learn about the allegations of abuse and feared that he would never see his daughter again. He was also concerned that his daughter might develop psychological problems due to allegations in the future.

Special Issues in Child Custody

Evaluators of child custody are requested to make recommendations on joint or sole custody and visitation schedules (Goldstein 2014). The evaluators are also requested to recommend on whether a "supervised visitation" with the child is necessary. The cases that are related to allegations of physical or sexual abuse, neglect, domestic violence; mental illness, and substance abuse may be evaluated in terms of a "supervised visitation" (Goldstein 2014). When the evaluators don't have the required training to assess these special issues, a consultant may be involved (Goldstein 2014; Baštecká and Boukalová 2020).

Assessments of sexual abuse and domestic violence allegations require a specialized evaluation (Goldstein 2014). It is reported that less than 50 percent of the sexual abuse allegations are substantiated (Bala et al. 2007). This ratio clarifies why a specialized assessment is needed.

Parental alienation cases also require a specialized evaluation. A child's strong preference for one parent does not always indicate purposeful indoctrination. There may be several reasons why a child prefers to be close to one parent and rejects visitation with the other parent. Maltreatment of the child, purposeful indoctrination, and accidental indoctrination (e.g., by an anxious parent) and children who are anxious, stubborn, or trying to escape conflict can be counted among the causes (Bernet 2002).

It is also important to emphasize that case-based assessment is essential while working with forensic cases since every case has a diverse history and different details. The experience of the evaluator is cumulative, but the assessment is case based. In the case illustration above, the possibility of an actual child abuse, the mother's motivation about these allegations and the risk for parental alienation should be kept in mind during the assessment.

Long-distance parenting, relocation, children with special needs, grandparents' rights, same-sex divorce, parental kidnapping, and nontraditional religious practices are among other special issues that may require recommendations from the evaluators (Goldstein 2014; Mroczkowski 2018).

Report Writing

The convictions of the evaluator should be based on information and data obtained by the implementation of reliable principles and methods (Martindale et al. 2007). Prior to writing the report, the evaluator should contemplate how the various outcomes might affect the family (Herman 1997). A simple and clear language should be used while writing the reports (Rohrbaugh 2008). The evaluator should refrain from using medical jargon in the reports (Herman 1997) since the readers will be judges and attorneys. If it is necessary to use medical terms, they must be defined (Kraus and Thomas 2011). It is essential to provide the information requested by the decision makers (Rohrbaugh 2008). Judges and attorneys expect a brief, child-focused, and objective report that includes information about the child, the strengths and weaknesses of the parents, and recommendations for custody and visitation (Bow and Quinnell 2004).

The child custody evaluation report should include the following subheadings (Bernet 2002):

1. Identifying information: Names and birthdates of the children and sides in competition (usually the parents).
2. Referral information: A brief history of the marriage, the current status of the children's custody and visitation, and a quotation from the court order that authorizes the evaluation, the conditions of the referral, and the specific aim of the evaluation.
3. Procedure for the evaluation: List of the interviews, the psychometric and psychological tests, and the collateral information.
4. Observations: Each parent is discussed separately, including strengths, weaknesses, personality traits, important medical and psychiatric problems, and whether these factors have a negative effect on the person's parenting abilities. Each child is discussed individually, including strengths and weaknesses, presence of any psychiatric disorder, and a remark about how the child is coping with the divorce. The child's attachment to each parent, the child's preference regarding custody and the reasons for the preference, and whether one of the parents has any undesirable effects on the child.
5. Conclusions: A list of specific statements that the evaluator thinks are supported by the data. For example, a parent's psychiatric disorder may affect his or her behavior toward the children.
6. Recommendations: The evaluator may recommend on the custody of the children, the visitation schedule, the need for supervised

visitation, psychiatric outpatient follow-up for any of the family members, and counseling for parenting.

CONCLUSION

Divorce is a process that includes not only couples but the whole family, especially children. In these cases, the forensic evaluation by a mental health professional is different from performing therapy. Child custody evaluation is a comprehensive process that includes having both knowledge about clinical aspects such as child and adolescent developmental issues and information about related ethical and legal issues. The evaluation is composed of interviews with parents, children, and other related people. Evaluators are required to assess factors related to the best interests of the child and need to look at special issues such as cases that are related to allegations of physical or sexual abuse, neglect, domestic violence, mental illness, and substance abuse.

REFERENCES

Achenbach, T. M. (1991). *Manual for the child behavior check-list/4-18 and 1991 profile*. Burlington (VT): University of Vermont Department of Psychiatry.

Ackerman, M. (1994). *Clinicians Guide to Child Custody Evaluations*. New York: Wiley.

Ackerman, M. J., Schoendorf, K. (1994). *ASPECT: Ackerman-Schoendorf scales for parent evaluation of custody*. Los Angeles: Western Psychological Services.

Amato, P. R. and Keith, B. (1991). Parental divorce and the well-being of children: a meta-analysis. *Psychological Bulletin*, 110, 26-46.

American Academy of Matrimonial Lawyer. (2013). Child custody evaluation standard. *Journal of American Academy of Matrimonial Law,* 25, 251-294.

American Psychological Association. (1995). Guidelines for child custody evaluations in divorce proceedings. *Family Law Q*, 29, 51-62.

Association of Family and Conciliation Courts. (1994). Association of Family and Conciliation Courts model standards of practice for child custody evaluation. *Family Court Review*, 32, 504-513.

Bala, N. M., Mitnick, M., Trocmé, N., Houston, C. (2007). Sexual abuse allegations and parental separation: smokescreen or fire? *Journal of Child and Family Studies,* 13, 26-56.

Barnum, R. (1987). Understanding controversies in visitation. *Journal of the American Academy of Child and Adolescent Psychiatry*, 26, 788-92.

Baštecká, B., Boukalová, H. (2020). Ethical Issues of Psychological Expert Testimony in Child Custody Cases: A Comparison of Ethical Approaches. *Psychology in Russia: State of the Art,* 13, 82-98.

Bene, E. (1985). *Family relations test: children's version.* Windsor, England: NFER-NELSON.

Benedek, R. S. and Benedek, E. P. (1980). Participating in child custody cases. In Chetky D. H. and Benedek E. P. (Eds) *Child Psychiatry and the Law*. S New York: Brunner/Mazel.

Benedek, E. P. and Schetky, D. H. (1985). Custody and visitation - perspectives. *Psychiatric Clinics of North America*, 8, 857-873.

Bernet, W. (1983). The therapist's role in child custody disputes. *Journal of American Academy Child Psychiatry*, 22, 180-183.

Bernet, W. (2002). Child custody evaluations. *Child and Adolescent Psychiatric Clinics of North America*, 11, 781-804.

Bow, J. N. and Quinell, F. A. (2002). A critical review of child custody evaluation reports. *Family Court Review*, 40, 164-176.

Bow, J. and Quinnell, F. A. (2004). Critique of child custody evaluations by the legal profession. *Family Court Review,* 42, 115-127.

Butcher, J. N., Graham, J. R., Dahlstrom, W. G. and Bowman, E. (1989). *Manual for administration and scoring: MMPI-2 (Minnesota*

Multiphasic Personality Inventory-2). Minneapolis: University of Minnesota Press.

Chung, D. S., Moon, D. S., Lee, M. H. and Kwack Y. S. (2020). Child Custody Evaluation Process and Report Writing. *Journal of Korean Academy of Child and Adolescent Psychiatry*, 31(2), 58-65.

Derdeyn, A. P. (1976). Child custody conflicts in historic perspective. *American Journal of Psychiatry* 133, 1369-1376.

Garner, R. A. (1991). *Psychotherapy with children of divorce*. Northvale (NJ): Jason Aronson Inc.

Goldstein, M. L. (2014). Child Custody Evaluations. In S. J. Morewitz and M. L. Goldstein (Eds.), *Handbook of Forensic Sociology and Psychology*, (pp. 305-321). doi: 10.1007/978-1-4614-7178-3_22, © Springer Science+Business Media New York.

Gould, J. W. (1998). *Conducting scientifically crafted child custody evaluations*. Thousand Oaks, CA: Sage Publications.

Haller, L. H. (1981). Before the judge: the child custody evaluation. *Adolescent Psychiatry*, 9, 142-164.

Heilburn, K. (1992). The role of psychological testing in forensic assessment. *Law and Human Behavior*, 16, 257-272.

Herman, S. P. (1997). Practice parameters for child custody evaluation. *Journal of the American Academy of Child and Adolescent Psychiatry*, 36(10), 57S-68S.

Howell, S. H., Portes, P. R and Brown, J. H. (1997). Gender and Age Differences in Child Adjustment to Parental Separation. *Journal of Divorce and Remarriage*, 27 (3/4), 141-158.

Kraus, L. J and Thomas, C. R. (2011). Practice parameter for child and adolescent forensic evaluations. *Journal of American Academy of Child and Adolescent Psychiatry*, 50, 1299-1312.

Lachar, D. (1999). *Personality Inventory for Children (PIC): revised format manual supplement.* Los Angeles: Western Psychological Services.

Lubit, R. (2005). Child Custody Evaluations. In K. Cheng and K. Myers (Eds.) *Child and Adolescent Psychiatry: The Essentials* (pp.381-395). Lippincott Williams & Wilkins.

Marlow, L. and Sauber, S. R. (1990). *The handbook of divorce mediation.* New York: Plenum Press.

Martindale, D. A., Martin, I., Auistin, W. G., Drozd, I., Gould-Saltman, D., Kirkpatrick, H. D., et al. (2007). Model standards of practice for child custody evaluation. *Family Court Review*, 45, 70-91.

Morey, L. C. (1991). *The personality assessment inventory professional manual*. Odessa (FL): psychological Assessment Resources.

Mroczkowski, M. M. (2018). Divorce and child custody. In A. Martin, M. Bloch & F. Volkmar (Eds.) *Lewis's Child and Adolescent Psychiatry: A Comprehensive Textbook.* Fifth Edition (pp. 2731-2936). Philadelphia: Wolters Kluwer.

Nurcombe, B. and Parlett, D. J. (1994). Child Custody Disputes. In: *Child mental health and the law*. New York: Free Press, 87-131.

OECD (The Organisation for Economic Co-operation and Development) Family Database. (2019). Retrieved November 14, 2020, from HYPERLINK "http://www.oecd.org/els/family/database.htm "http://www.oecd.org/els/family/database.htm.

Rohrbaugh, J. B. (2008). Writing the Report. *A comprehensive guide to child custody evaluations: Mental health and legal perspectives.* (pp. 323-348). Springer Science + Business Media. HYPERLINK "https://psycnet.apa.org/doi/10.1007/978-0-387-71894-1" https://doi.org/10.1007/978-0-387-71894-1.

Saposnek, D. T. (1998). *Mediating child custody disputes: a strategic approach.* San Francisco: Jossey-Bass.

United Nations, Department of Economic and Social Affairs, Population Division. (2019). Retrieved November 14, 2020, from https://population.un.org/MarriageData/Index.html#/maritalStatusChart.

US Commission on Child and Family Welfare. (1996). *Parenting our children: in the best interest of the nation: a report to the President and congress*. Washington, DC.

Weithorn, L. A. (1987). *Psychology and Child Custody Determinations.* Lincoln: University of Nebraska.

In: Forensic Psychiatry …
Editor: Nursen Turan Yurtsever
ISBN: 978-1-53619-530-9

Chapter 10

CHILD AND ADOLESCENT PSYCHIATRY PERSPECTIVE IN FORENSIC CASES

Aliye Tugba Bahadir*
Marmara University School of Medicine, Department of Child & Adolescent Psychiatry, Istanbul, Turkey

ABSTRACT

Forensic assessment of children and adolescents is an important and specialized area in child and adolescent psychiatry. Nearly every child and adolescent psychiatrist or other professional working with children and adolescents is requested to assess forensic cases and is expected to write objective forensic reports with clear language. A multidisciplinary approach helps to reach a more integrative perspective and to identify blurry points in the cases, thereby contributing to the quality of the evaluation. Child maltreatment may affect all domains of development and may have short and long term adverse effects on mental and physical health. Maltreatment can also negatively affect the development of a secure attachment between the child and his/her primary caregivers, and may jeopardize the ability to build healthy relationships throughout life. Therefore, recognizing abuse and neglect, reducing the risk, increasing

* Corresponding Author's E-mail: tugba772004@yahoo.com.

resilience, and helping to reach the best possible outcome for the child/adolescent are important in terms of the approach to maltreatment. Therefore I would like to describe the key points related to the interview of forensic cases, highlight the facilitating and attention requiring aspects in the evaluation, and reflect on the perspective of child and adolescent psychiatry.

INTRODUCTION

Evaluation of child and adolescent forensic cases has some key points that can facilitate the process. This chapter provides guidance particularly for child and adolescent psychiatrists and also a broad range of other professionals who are involved in children's mental health would benefit from this manuscript. Throughout this chapter the term 'interviewer' is used to indicate a child and adolescent psychiatrist or other child mental health professional who evaluates child and adolescent forensic cases.

STEPWISE INTERVIEW FOR FORENSIC EVALUATION

A step by step interview was described by Yuille et al., (1993) (cited in Bernet 1997). This systematic interview style is useful for obtaining salient information related to abused children.

Building Rapport

In some cases, two or three interviews may be required for building rapport. While building a good relationship with the child or adolescent, the interviewer observes the child's cognitive and social skills and behavior. Moreover, how can someone expect a child to tell about a traumatic event in a context when the sense of connection has not yet been built?

Explaining Two Specific Events

The interviewer requests the child to describe two events in the past, such as a birthday party. These non-leading and open-ended questions serve as a model for the rest of the interview for the child.

Telling the Truth

The interviewer states the necessity of only telling the truth during the interview. The interviewer starts with general questions and continues with specific questions if needed.

Introducing the Subject of Concern

Again the interviewer may start from general questions and continue with specific questions. "Do you know why we are talking today?", "Has anyone done anything to you?" Drawings may also be helpful in initiating the disclosure of the event.

Free Narrative

The interviewer requests the child to describe the events from the beginning including all the details. The child continues to tell at his/her own pace. If the abuse happened over a long time period, the interviewer may first request a description of the general pattern of the events and afterwards may ask for specific incidents.

General Questions

The interviewer may ask general questions to elucidate additional details. The questions should not be leading, such as "Your father's friend touched your legs, didn't he?" or suggestive such as "Did your father's friend touch your legs?"

Specific Questions

The interviewer may want to clarify some issues by asking more specific questions, particularly when trying to elucidate inconsistencies in a gentle way.

If the child uses an age inappropriate word, the interviewer may ask where he/she learned the word. The interviewer should avoid asking repetitive questions, and also should avoid rewarding and praising answers.

Using Interview Aids, If Needed

Anatomical dolls may be beneficial for clarifying the type of abusive act that had happened. They are used for the elucidation of the event, not for diagnostic purposes.

Concluding the Interview

The interviewer may ask a few leading questions about unrelated topics, to have an idea about the susceptibility of the child. A question like 'You came to the hospital by bus, didn't you?' may be asked to reveal the suggestibility of the child. If the child displays susceptibility to suggestions, the interviewer would need to confirm that the previous information obtained is reliable and not contaminated. The interviewer concludes the interview by thanking the child. The interviewer should not make any promises that he/she can't keep.

Additionally, ending the interview with a positive topic is also important (Lobel 2014), since talking about traumatic events would be stressful for the child.

Table 1. below is a summary of don't's during the assessment (Bernet 1997).

Table 1. What to avoid during the assessment

Avoid making multiple assessments if you can
Avoid asking leading and suggestive questions
Avoid asking repetitive or multiple questions or long questions that have or's/and's in them
Avoid reacting to inconsistencies in a threatening manner
Avoid rewarding answers, particularly with praise
Avoid making any promises that you can't keep

Conditions Preventing the Child from Explaining the Abuse History

One of the most important points in forensic psychiatric assessment of children and adolescents is that they may hide information or they may tell information that is not true because of the pressure from adults in their environment (Bernet 1993, Bernet 1997). Threats of the perpetrators may create fear and prevent the child/adolescent from telling the abuse history.

The child's age may be too young to tell a story (Guerra et al., 2012) that describes the flow of events. For children and adolescents in a manic or mixed episode of bipolar disorder (Marvel and Paradiso 2004) or in a psychotic episode (Otgaar et al., 2017) recalling problems; for children and adolescents with mental retardation problems with comprehension may present a challenge in terms of explaining the abuse history accurately.

Communication problems, mental retardation and autism would obviously cause problems in explaining the abuse.

What Do We Do When It's Difficult to Learn the Abuse History or When Everything Is Not Clear Enough?

Besides the child or adolescent and the parents, receiving information from multiple informants such as teachers and relatives (if they know the event), regarding the behavioral and emotional changes after the abuse/neglect period is very valuable. But the interviewer should be careful to not inform a teacher or a relative who does not know about the abuse.

If the interviewer has concerns of the accuracy of information he/she received, it is always better to consult the forensic psychiatry department and schedule another interview with the child and the family and pay close attention to any inconsistencies related to how the child/family describe the events generally and evaluate the psyhiatric symptoms again.

When facts are not clear enough, the child and adolescent psychiatrists and forensic medicine experts can hold multidisciplinary meetings to contemplate whether the event really happened or not. The nature of the way events happen may attract the evaluators' attention to cases that are not clear. Is the way events occured coherent with the normal course of life? This is an important question to spot blurry and inconsistent points in a forensic case.

What Is Important? What Do We Pay Attention To During the Psychiatric Assessment?

Once the interviewer has a strong opinion that the event has happened, afterwards more attention can be allocated to making the psychiatric diagnoses. Besides the emotional and behavioral information received in the forensic evaluation, the child and adolescent psychiatrist now has the opportunity to deepen the psychiatric assessment.

Emotional and behavioral status before and after the event and emotional and behavioral changes before and after the event are important. Some changes may be irrelevant to the (abusive) event, such as adjustment problems due to divorce of the parents. In case of the presence of more than one event, the child and adolescent psychiatrist should try to clarify these emotional and behavioral states and changes before and after each event.

It is very important to make an accurate diagnosis. The interview is supported by psychiatric rating scales and psychometric tests, and projective tests when required. Taking notes adequately in the patient file is essential for a child and adolescent psychiatrist. It is a requirement of professional work and would also be very helpful for further judicial requests of the patient files, since any case can become a forensic case in time. It is also important to highlight here that the reporting of child maltreatment cases is required by law (Kaufman and Hoover 2018).

For Both the Abuse History and Psychiatric Assessment We Pay Attention to the Following

Consistency

Inconsistency should attract the attention of the interviewer (O'Donohue et al., 2010). Consistency within the story and consistency within and between the informants is important while assessing forensic cases. When there is inconsistency between the child/adolescent and one of the parents/relatives, the interviewer should be cautious about the possibility that one of the informants may be trying to hide the truth.

Statements Inappropriate for Developmental Stage

When a child composes a complex sentence including a comment or information that is unlikely for them to express or know at his/her age, the interviewer should keep in mind that this expression may have been taught by someone else (Bernet 1997).

Attitude Towards the Interviewer/Assessment/ Psychometric Testing

This gives clues regarding the intention of the child or adolescent and/or the family. If hostile attitude is present towards the interviewer or the psychologist who implements the psychometric tests, the interviewer should be cautious about the possibility of hidden information.

Behavioral Indicators, Psychological and Psychiatric Consequences of Child Maltreatment

The maltreated child may display the following behaviors:

Table 2. Possible Behavioral Indicators of Abuse (Al Odhayani et al., 2013)

1-Displays unusual agression
2-Startles when touched
3-Changes in school performance and attendance
4-Draws back from family and friends
5-Uninterested in activities previously enjoyed
5-Low self-esteem
6-Suicidal thoughts or self-destructive behaviors
7-Displays risky behaviors
8-Engages in age-inappropriate sexual play

Table 3. Possible Behavioral Indicators of Neglect (Al Odhayani et al., 2013)

1-Developmental delay related to lack of stimulation
2-Problems related to attention and school attendance
3-Takes on a caregiver role for a parent or siblings
4-Appears unhappy or has flat affect
5-Lack of energy
6-Unwilling to go home, speaks of being alone at home

Psychological Effects of Child Abuse and Neglect (Cicchetti and Toth 1995)

1. Affect dysregulation
2. Disruptive and aggressive behaviors
3. Insecure attachment
4. Spoiled peer relationships with increased aggression or social withdrawal
5. Academic underachievement
6. Low self-esteem
7. Various psychopathologies

Psychiatric Diagnoses Related to Child Maltreatment

Child maltreatment is a risk factor for the development of psychopathology (Childers 2005). The following psychiatric symptoms and diagnoses are more frequently encountered in maltreated children than the community controls (Kaufman and Hoover 2018).

1. Externalizing and internalizing behavior problems
2. Posttraumatic stress disorder

3. Depression
4. Reactive attachment disorder and disinhibited social engagement disorder
5. Dissociative symptoms
6. Suicidality, self-destructive behavior, borderline traits
7. Drug and alcohol problems
8. Eating disorders
9. Oppositional defiant disorder
10. Conduct disorder and development of sociopathy later in life

Case 1

Gülfidan is a 16 year-old girl who was admitted to the emergency service due to attempting suicide with her mother's anti-hypertensive drugs and pain killers she had found at home. After the initial treatment at the emergency service, it turned out that the reason for her suicide attempt was ongoing abuse from her father. She said 'I can't take this anymore.' The adolescent stated that the abuse was going on since she was 13 years old. At the interview with the mother, she was in denial and she claimed that her daughter was making this claim because her father didn't let her see her boyfriend. The child psychiatrist handled the inconsistent information very carefully so that the adolescent and mother would not be scared and withdraw from the assessment and further treatment process. The case was reported to the judicial authorities. It took some time, but with close follow-up in the adult psychiatry outpatient clinic, the mother accepted the reality of abuse. In the follow-up period the adolescent's suicidal thoughts decreased.

As described in the case above, the underlying reason behind suicide attempts may sometimes be abuse history.

Recognize **R**educe the **R**isk Increase **R**esilience Help to **R**each the best possible among multiple outcomes for the child

CONCLUSION

Childhood and adolescence is clearly an important period which has the potential to affect the course of life in a substantial way. It is a period that includes development in which biological and psychosocial components are at interaction and therefore has both opportunities and risks. Various outcomes are possible for every child and adolescent. The role of the child and adolescent mental health professional is to help the child to be in the best possible state mentally and emotionally, regardless of past adverse experiences. This would contribute to a better future for all.

> "If I can stop one heart from breaking,
> I shall not live in vain;
> If I can ease one life the aching,
> Or cool one pain,
> Or help one fainting robin unto his nest again,
> I shall not live in vain."
> Emily Dickinson

REFERENCES

Al Odhayani, A., Watson, W. J., Watson, L. (2013). Behavioural consequences of child abuse. *Canadian Family Physician*, 59, 831-836.

Bernet, W. (1993). False statements and the differential diagnosis of abuse allegations. *Journal of the American Academy of Child and Adolescent Psychiatry*, 32, 903-910.

Bernet, W. (1997). Practice Parameters for the Forensic Evaluation of Children and Adolescents Who May Have Been Physically or Sexually Abused. *Journal of the American Academy of Child and Adolescent Psychiatry,* 36, 37S-56S.

Childers, A. M. (2005). In K. Cheng and K. Myers (Eds.) *Child and Adolescent Psychiatry: The Essentials*. (pp. 363-379) Philadelphia: Lippincott Williams & Wilkins.

Cicchetti, D., Toth, S. L. (1995). A developmental psychopathology perspective on child abuse and neglect. *Journal of the American Academy of Child and Adolescent Psychiatry*, 34,541-565.

Guerra, N., Williamson, A., Lucas-Molina, Beatriz. (2012). Normal development: Infancy, childhood, and adolescence. In Rey J.M. (Ed). *International Handbook of Child and Adolescent Mental Health* (pp.1-39). International Association for Child and Adolescent Psychiatry and Allied Professions. Retrieved from: https://iacapap.org/content/uploads/A.2.-DEVELOPMENT-072012.pdf.

Kaufman, J., Hoover, D. (2018). Child Abuse and Neglect. In A. Martin, M. Bloch & F. Volkmar (Eds.) *Lewis's Child and Adolescent Psychiatry: A Comprehensive Textbook.* Fifth Edition (pp.644-651). Philadelphia: Wolters Kluwer.

Lobel, D. S. (2014). Forensic Evaluation of Child Abuse. In S. J. Morewitz and M. L. Goldstein (Eds.), *Handbook of Forensic Sociology and Psychology*, (pp. 363-374). DOI 10.1007/978-1-4614-7178-3_22, © Springer Science+Business Media New York.

Marvel, C. L., Paradiso, S. (2004). Cognitive and neurological impairment in mood disorders. *Psychiatry Clinics of North America*, 27, 19-36.

O'Donohue, W., Benuto, L., Fanetti M. (2010). Children's Allegations of Sexual Abuse: A Model for Forensic Assessment. *Psychological Injury and Law*, 3,148-154.

Otgaar, H., Muris, P., Howe, M. L., Merckelbach, H. (2017). What Drives False Memories in Psychopathology? A Case for Associative Activation. *Clinical Psychological Science*, 5,1048–1069.

ABOUT THE EDITOR

Nursen Turan Yurtsever was born on 25 July 1971 in Istanbul, in Turkey. After graduating from the Istanbul University, Cerrahpasa Medical School in 1995, she specialized in Forensic Medicine at the Council of Forensic Medicine, Turkey in 2003. Turan Yurtsever has been an Associated Professor of Forensic Medicine (2012 to 2021). While working at Karadeniz Technical University, Trabzon, Turkey (2006 to 2014), she established the Institute of Forensic Sciences at Karadeniz Technical University in 2013 and Child Protection Center at Karadeniz Technical University in 2014. She studied and presented lectures at the Forensic Institute of Coimbra University, Portugal in 2008 and at the Medical Examiner Office of Tarrant County, Texas, USA in 2011. She is still the clinical manager of Forensic Medicine Department of Pendik Education and Research Hospital at Marmara University, and Pendik Child Protection Centre, in Istanbul, Turkey. Her field of study is on Forensic Psychiatry, Human Rights, Child Abuse and Neglect, and Clinical Forensic Medicine. She is author of over 50 peer reviewed publications, 40 conference presentations, 5 book chapters and advisor of many thesis, and research projects about Forensic Psychiatry, Human Rights, Child Abuse and Neglect, and Forensic Medicine.

INDEX

A

D

E

M

R

S

W

Y